Fighting
Drug Abuse With
Acupuncture

Fighting Drug Abuse With Acupuncture: The Treatment That Works

Ellinor R. Mitchell

Pacific View Press
Berkeley, CA

Library of Congress Catalog Card Number 95-69800
ISBN 1-881896-12-9

Printed in the United States of America

Quotations from *Banks of Marble*, words and music by
Les Rice, ©1950, Stormking Music, Inc., appear in this book.

To Ray Gordon who,
as always, enhances the journey.

CONTENTS

PREFACE

The American public was jolted into awareness of acupuncture on July 26, 1971, when *New York Times* Senior Editor James Reston published an account of his appendectomy in Beijing.

"The facts are," Reston wrote, "that with the assistance of eleven of the leading medical specialists in Peking, who were asked by Premier Chou En-lai to cooperate on the case, Prof. Wu Wei-jan of the Anti-Imperialist Hospital's* surgical staff removed my appendix on July 17 after a normal injection of Xylocain and Benzocain, which anesthetized the middle of my body.

"There were no complications, nausea or vomiting.

"I was conscious throughout, followed the instructions of Professor Wu as translated to me by Ma Yu-chen of the Chinese Foreign Ministry during the operation, and was back in my bedroom in the hospital in two and a half hours.

"However, I was in considerable discomfort if not pain during the second night after the operation, and Li Chang-yuan, doctor of acupuncture at the hospital, with my approval, inserted three long, thin needles into the outer part of my right elbow and below my knees and manipulated them in order to stimulate the intestine and release the pressure and distension of the stomach.

"That sent ripples of pain racing through my limbs and, at least, had the effect of diverting my attention from the distress in my stomach. Meanwhile, Doctor Li lit two pieces of an herb called *ai,* which looked like the burning stumps of a broken cheap cigar, and held them close to my abdomen while occasionally twirling the needles into action.

"All this took about 20 minutes, during which I remember thinking that it was rather a complicated way to get rid of gas on the stomach, but there was a noticeable relaxation of the pressure and distension within an hour and no recurrence of the problem thereafter."

Reston went on to describe the collaboration between the MD and the acupuncturist in that Chinese hospital.

"Dr. Li Chang-yuan, who used needle and herbal medicine on me, did not go to medical college. He . . . learned his craft as an apprentice to a veteran acupuncturist here at the hospital.

The other doctors watched him . . . with obvious respect. Prof. Li Pang-chi said later that he had not been a believer in the use of acupuncture techniques, 'but a fact is a fact—there are many things they can do.' "

Prof. Chen Hsien-jiu of the hospital's surgery department told Reston that he had studied the effects of acupuncture in overcoming postoperative constipation by putting barium in a patient's stomach and observing on a fluoroscope how needle manipulation in the limbs produced movement and relief in the intestines.

It is worth noting that the MD's in Reston's account worked respectfully with the acupuncturist, that the MD's skepticism was tempered by intellectual willingness to accept acupuncture's evident effectiveness, and that the Chinese surgeon had used Western scientific methods to investigate a specific acupuncture effect. In a modern Western-medicine hospital, setting Reston was treated with traditional Chinese medicine, whose diagnostic and therapeutic techniques have endured for more than 2,000 years.

Acupuncture is part of Chinese traditional medicine, whose other therapies include herbalism, diet, exercise and massage. From a simple form recorded in China around 1500 B.C.E., acupuncture developed into a regular system with repeatable results which were classified and described by 200 B.C.E. By the middle of the sixth century C.E., Chinese medicine was practiced in Korea and Japan. Chinese acupuncture texts and commentaries, and their translations, were indispensable to the spread of this medical practice throughout China's sphere of influence. Since the 17th century, interest in acupuncture has washed in and out of the Occident on tides of commerce and diplomacy. For more than 300 years acupuncture has been discussed, tried, ignored, scorned, re-examined, dismissed, rediscovered, studied and practiced in the West.

Acupuncturists diagnose and treat illness, and relieve pain, by sticking fine solid needles into specific points on the body, head, arms and legs. Acupuncture stimulates the body's natural tendency to resist or overcome ailments. In ways still not fully understood, it also prompts a biochemical response that decreases or eliminates painful sensations. By practice and theory it has evolved into a complete system of effective treatment for many illnesses, and for injuries which do not require prompt surgery.

Acupuncture has been adjusted to meet patients' needs in different eras and in different societies, and new methods continue to be developed in China and other countries to augment ancient techniques. In China, where Western medicine had been taught since 1835, the decade of the 1950s marked a great shaking up of acupuncture's centuries-old techniques and applications. "Health care for all the people" was a stated goal of Mao Zedong's revolution. The central government decreed that the 70,000 doctors trained in Western medicine and the 500,000 trained in traditional Chinese medicine must learn from each other. This mandate resulted in the development by 1957 of acupuncture-anesthesia (technically *analgesia,* as the patient remains conscious) for use in major surgery; as well as advances in electroacupuncture; and initiation of research to explain acupuncture in terms of Western medicine.

Innovations since 1957 include the use of low-voltage electroacupuncture, laser acupuncture and injection of Western medications at acupuncture points, a procedure which can lessen the amount of medication required for effective treatment.

Needles are manipulated to modify their effect, and for some conditions practitioners now apply electrostimulation: wires from an electrical output device with a range of frequencies and impulses are clipped to inserted needles. Instead of using needles, some acupuncturists set flat electrodes directly on acupuncture points.

Ear acupuncture, electroacupuncture and veterinary acupuncture (applied to domestic animals in China as early as the 14th century) were practiced and became subjects of continuing research in England, France, Germany and Italy long before American scientists undertook substantial investigation. The United States is the last major Western nation to take acupuncture seriously. In the past twenty years the extent of acupuncture practice and the establishment of professional acupuncture associations have paved the way for collaboration between acupuncturists and US health-care institutions.

A distinctly American adaptation of acupuncture, developed at the drug clinic of Lincoln Hospital in New York's South Bronx and disseminated by the National Acupuncture Detoxification Association (NADA), has made a major contribution to health care in the treatment of drug addiction. This is a health problem whose financial and social costs extend far beyond the plight of the individual addict.

---

*This hospital, established in 1916 as the Peking Union Medical College, funded by the Rockefeller Foundation, built and run by the China Medical Board of New York, was nationalized in 1951.

ACKNOWLEDGEMENTS

Above all, thanks are due to staff at clinics where I observed the use of acupuncture in addiction treatment. Special thanks to the acupuncturists and detox specialists who allowed me to receive treatment alongside clients, whose friendliness enlivened the experience.

People named and unnamed in the book generously gave time and energy to interviews. Their patience recalled the venerable teaching slogan, "There are no stupid questions."

My special gratitude to Mike Smith, who opened doors, including the one to an illuminating staff discussion of Lincoln Acupuncture Clinic's early days.

I am indebted to Carlos Alvarez for archival help and for his continual willingness to clarify my impressions about Lincoln and NADA.

Thanks also to Yoshiaki Omura for insights and professional hospitality; to Ron Rosen for long-distance comradeship; and to Wei-Ming Tsao for consultation during the process of writing this book.

Others who graciously informed me, while present in memory are no longer here to read my appreciation: Carlos Aponte, Carole Myers, Father Mark Pemberton, and Paul Zmiewski.

Many people outside the acupuncture community contributed to this book. Among them, family and friends whose provocative questions helped me avoid false assumptions.

I am also grateful for the diligent editorial support of Pacific View Press.

Contributions to this view of how acupuncture-based addiction treatment took root and flourished in the United States came from many sources; but the author is accountable for any misconceptions.

1

ACUPUNCTURE
AND ADDICTION TREATMENT

We foot the bill for substance abuse—whether we allocate tax dollars to healing, which in the process of change offers hope, or to building more prisons which simply warehouse addicts until they are released to pursue the same old life and do not change drug-seeking behavior.

The misery shared by millions of addicts, their families and their friends cannot be quantified, only experienced or observed. Addiction's cost to society, however, *can* be calculated: The price for substance abuse—the term coined years ago to describe addiction to both illegal and legal drugs—is $237.5 billion per year, according to an estimate published by the Robert Wood Johnson Foundation (*Substance Abuse: The Nation's Number One Health Problem*).

The Johnson Foundation report assigns $66.9 billion of the annual $237.5 billion pricetag to drug abuse, $98.6 billion to alcohol abuse and $72 billion to smoking. The report estimates that substance-abuse-related expenses—costs which would not be incurred were it not for addiction's daunting prevalence—equal $1,000 per year taken from every man, woman and child in this country.

Some $34 billion of this bill goes to health care: as the report says, "A heavy smoker will stay 25 percent longer when hospitalized than a nonsmoker, a problem drinker four times as long as a nondrinker." And there are more direct links. HIV-disease is spread by intravenous-drug users sharing contaminated needles; neonatal intensive hospital care for drug-affected newborns ranges from $40,000 to over $100,000 per patient. These are just two examples.

Addiction affects manufacturing and commerce. Fifty-five percent of the 6 million illicit-drug users in the United States are employed, as are most smokers and many alcoholics. The impaired work performance and health problems of all three groups raise the cost of goods and services just as shoplifting raises retail prices.

Drug addiction contaminates housing and neighborhoods and decreases public safety; it erodes education and increases the demand for social services.

Drug addiction is a major cost factor in the criminal justice system, from arrest through the judicial process to incarceration. Seventy to 80 percent of arrestees test positive for drugs. Fifty percent of the men arrested for homicide and violent assault test positive for drugs.

Of the more than one million people serving time in our constantly expanding federal and state prison systems, at least 30 percent are incarcerated because of involvement with drugs. This alone costs nearly $10 billion annually. In Florida it costs $15,000 to $17,000 per year to keep an inmate in the county jail. Room and board and tuition in the state penitentiary—what some experts call the college-level correctional institution—is $30,000 per year per inmate. At New York's Rikers Island it costs $58,000 to maintain one prisoner for one year. (It costs $31,365 to keep a residential student for a year at Barnard, a private college of Columbia University in nearby Manhattan.) New York State alone spends $3 billion a year on prisons whose population has increased 500 percent in 20 years.

The cost of expanding the prison system to contain ever greater numbers of drug offenders—figured at $100,000 per bed for new construction—is likely to surge now that two states, Washington and California, have adopted "three strikes and you're out" laws, mandating life imprisonment without possibility of parole for defendants convicted of their third separate violent felony. California's state budget increased its allocations to the penal system by almost 10 percent after passage of the law, bringing expenditures to almost $4 billion in that state alone.

Treatment for illegal drug use and alcoholism has existed for decades, but still it is neither plentiful nor always attractive to clients. The prevailing national estimate is that conventional treatment—therapeutic communities and hospital inpatient or outpatient services, among other settings—serves one addict in four.

In the last decade $14 billion has been spent on high-tech, high-cost approaches to cutting the drug supply, to no effect. Low-tech but definitely high-cost imprisonment—for the most part, with very little treatment available—has not deterred drug use and drug dealing.

But there does exist an innovative, low-cost, effective means of treating addiction to illegal drugs and to alcohol, the preeminent legal drug. This approach, using acupuncture, has a twenty-year track record and is gaining acceptance by agencies and institutions deeply frustrated by past failure. Three hundred health facilities in twenty states now provide drug-abuse treatment that uses acupuncture according to a therapeutic design originating at Lincoln Hospital in New York. Nine other countries have programs based on this method, which among other things uses ear-acupuncture, chamomile-based herbal tea and regular urine testing.

For too long, those who insist drug addiction is purely a crime to be punished have contended with those who see it as a disease to be treated. The experience of rehabilitating addicts by treating addiction as a disease rather than a crime discredits proposals to pour billions of dollars into the prison industry to punish people rather than help them recover. Acupuncture-based treatment works. Clinic by clinic it is supplanting the vindictive attitude of jail-builders and of those who purport to wage a "war" on drugs.

Since 1989 a court in Dade County, Florida has demonstrated the economic common sense and compassion of a therapeutic approach to coping with drug addicts arrested for nonviolent offenses. Of 6,000 people accepted into the program since it began, 3,480 have completed it; 1,200 are currently enrolled. Nationally, 60 percent of people arrested on drug charges are rearrested. But the rearrest rate for graduates of Dade County's drug court is under 40 percent.

By late 1994, of the more than 6,000 who had entered the Miami program, 72 percent stayed in treatment; 28 percent either dropped out or were rearrested and dismissed from the program. Dade's Diversion and Treatment Program costs out at $500 to $750 per participant per year— less than 4 percent of the annual cost per inmate for imprisonment in Florida.

Miami's program is a leading example of acupuncture's practical power to keep nonviolent defendants *in* treatment and *out* of jail. The drug court's philosophy is finding increasing acceptance in the criminal justice system. By late 1993, eight other Florida counties—Broward, Escambia, Hillsborough, Lee, Leon, Monroe, Palm Beach, and Pinellas —had adopted the Dade County model. Nationwide, drug courts have been formed in Mobile, Alabama; Little Rock, Arkansas; St. Joseph, Michigan; Kansas City, Missouri; Las Vegas, Nevada; Portland, Oregon; and Austin and Beaumont, Texas. Acupuncture is integral to all these court-linked treatment programs.

The First National Drug Court Conference, held in Miami in December 1993, was funded by the National Institute of Justice and planned as a small working group to discuss drug court issues. This event attracted more than 400 people from all over the United States. Judges, defense lawyers, prosecutors and other members of the criminal justice community, as well as drug-treatment providers, were addressed by U.S. Attorney General Janet Reno. She noted the drug court movement's astonishing growth. Attendees observed Miami's drug court, and exchanged information about initiating and conducting similar venues—courts intimately involved in treatment of drug offenders.

Acupuncture-based addiction treatment, codified and disseminated by the National Acupuncture Detoxification Association (NADA), takes place in many different settings. Among them are community health clinics, court-affiliated programs in which defendants may choose treatment instead of incarceration, halfway houses, jails, prisons and a variety of other criminal justice facilities. Private mental health clinics employ the treatment as do methadone maintenance programs, municipal hospitals, Native American chemical-dependency clinics and counseling centers both urban and rural. Clients of acupuncture-based programs include adults and infants, people headed for jail and those already incarcerated, those whose chief distinguishing problem is addiction, and those for whom addiction is just one health disorder among many, including AIDS.

A typical effective and comprehensive yet inexpensive rehabilitation program combines acupuncture with group work such as 12-Step meetings and individual counseling. Programs of this type are being used successfully in the United States from New York's South Bronx to Indian reservations, and abroad from the slums of London through Western Europe and Hungary to Katmandu.

In South Dakota, acupuncture-based programs treat Native American alcoholics. A New York City clinic is helping to break the multigenerational cycle of child abuse in a program that combines acupuncture with comprehensive treatment of drug-using parents. Prisoners in Minnesota receive acupuncture for substance abuse problems. An acupuncture-based general clinic in Oregon also offers substance abuse treatment to its clients, some of whom are HIV-positive.

Acupuncture-based programs offer healing and thus hope to addicts and to their loved ones, who have said all too often, "He's finally getting it together, trying a new program," or, "This time she's been clean for a month; maybe she'll make it." Some people have, too often, been summoned to a hospital only to watch someone die. Acupuncture-based treatment is very good news for our drug-ridden society.

Experts on the drug plague say that treatment works. But as anyone who cares about an addicted person knows, it is often a struggle to get chemically dependent people into treatment and to retain them in a process that goes beyond detoxification to recovery and maintenance of recovery, and thereby changes their lives.

Some people enter addiction treatment voluntarily. Many are prodded by criminal justice and social service agencies to enroll in treatment programs as a condition of probation—a period of supervision in lieu of incarceration—or of parole—time after release from prison that completes the term of a sentence. For others, it is a condition for regaining child custody.

Industrial and office workers are candidates for cure, as are corporate CEOs. Addiction is an equal opportunity affliction. While the media repeatedly emphasize the problem of drugs in the black community—almost to the point of racist stereotyping—the fact is that addiction to drugs, both legal and illegal, pervades our whole society.

The candidate for cure is the guy on parole, in a job-skills program after eight years in prison for predicate felony—hurt an old man and only got chump change. Went cold turkey in the joint, came out clean, stayed that way for six months. Gets a job. Mom is living on workman's compensation, they can always use a little extra, the street has faster ways to make good money. Being around the stuff, a little taste can't hurt. Pretty soon he's nodding out on the couch watching TV and it doesn't take Moms too long to know it's not because the movie bores him. She won't kick him out, not yet, just cries when she looks at him. He won't last long on the job with the dealer if he comes up short for using too much product. One day when she's out of the house he'll sell the TV, and when she finds more of her stuff missing, even Moms won't hang in. Get straight, get employment—it's a steep climb or a slippery slide.

Another one's the woman who never does coke when she's down, only when she's feeling good and wants to pump up her exhilaration. Then she drops her calm executive-secretary façade, tells everyone what's wrong with their personalities and with how they conduct their lives, and makes more enemies than she has friends left. Her longtime lover, clean and sober for five years, has moved out again, for good.

And there is the young drifter who refuses to try Alcoholics Anonymous. Hits the 5 P.M. Happy Hour and calls it Attitude Adjustment. This is the third state he's lived in since dropping out of high school seven years ago. His driver's license has been suspended for Driving While Intoxicated. Eight months, this time. He's running out of friends who can drive him to pick up day jobs—or to the bar. Can't pay the rent. Last night he went to move his jeep to a neighbor's yard, and backed over his old black dog who screamed and howled and moaned before she died. Gotta get clean, try the army—or something.

And there is the heiress who has hit the ceiling again, spending $2,000 a month on heroin. That's when she always tapers down. "Can you believe it, my grandmother left me a million, and I'm down to a hundred thousand?" Ten years ago she put part of her inheritance into an irrevocable trust for her then-two-year-old's college education. Now she talks nonstop about how to break that money loose. "My daughter's cool, she understands I'm sick. When I stop being sick, I'm going to take a course, landscape gardening, you can make money in that." Fifteen years into a heavy habit. Fifteen years and ten fresh starts later, she remembers the pain of each withdrawal, and the vomiting. Maybe she can't quit, but she really must cut down.

Entering treatment is crucial. However, addicted people tend to drop out of treatment when they feel better, or when short-term goals are achieved. But recovery from addiction is long-term, which is why some groups, like Alcoholics Anonymous, regard it as a lifelong process.

Acupuncture detoxification is a gateway to recovery. Thousands of documented clinical cases show that drug-addicted patients like the effects of acupuncture. They say it calms the spirit, reduces cravings and alleviates tension, anxiety and dread. An acupuncture drug-treatment clinic, where many people sit in a treatment room with needles in their ears, is a tranquil place—most clients appear to be meditating. The atmosphere provides the luxury of peacefulness, a quality lacking in the life of anyone gripped by addiction.

Wherever it is practiced, the acupuncture-detoxification procedure is basically the same. You sit in a room with other clients and, like them, have three to five very fine acupuncture needles inserted at specific locations in the outer ear. The needles go under the skin, *not* through the ear. Any slight pain you might feel is fleeting. You've been through worse, or you wouldn't have come here. You sit and relax—yes! Relax.

What do you feel? The usual sensation is a release of tension—the insistent tension that obsessively repeats, "I need my fix," or "I gotta have a drink." Many acupuncture patients report, "It just feels like you've come home." Perhaps you will drift into meditation, or just sit watching your thoughts go by, maybe thinking about the last time you tried to kick, maybe wondering if you know the guy three chairs away. He looks familiar . . .

About 45 minutes later, the needles are removed. You may sit for a while before going back outside into the world. Either at the time of your admission, or after treatment, you receive tea bags containing an herbal mix which is nonnarcotic but helps you relax. You may drink a cup of this anytime, but must be sure to have some at bedtime. You feel better. You return the next day.

The procedures described here are becoming standard, but clinical variations do occur, as is often the case in conventional therapies.

Detox generally involves daily ear-acupuncture treatments. During this period you give a urine sample before each treatment. The sample is computer-analyzed: day by day you see a printout. When you have drugs in your system, the computer reports this on paper. Slipping isn't good, but everybody in the clinic knows it happens. When your printout shows ten consecutive clean urines, the next stage of the process begins: you continue to give urines and receive ear-acupuncture, while also participating in Narcotics Anonymous (NA) or Alcoholics Anonymous (AA), generally referred to as 12-Step groups.

Acupuncture-based programs *attract* addicted people by accepting walk-in clients as well as those referred by criminal justice or social service agencies, and by keeping intake paperwork to a minimum. They *retain* clients because acupuncture supports the hard work of becoming clean and sober, and of going on to engage in other elements of comprehensive treatment, including 12-Step work, prenatal care for pregnant addicts, group and individual counseling, men's groups, women's groups, educational and vocational placement, and other social services. Since it can be applied as needed to support a patient's recovery, acupuncture is the finest kind of insurance policy for chemically dependent people whose illness is characterized by relapse.

Acupuncture-based addiction treatment is a health-care bargain. It is a bargain for clients, many of whom have custody of children, go to school, and have jobs. (In 1990 William Bennett, federal "drug czar," said that "seventy percent of the regular drug users in the United States hold full-time jobs.") Outpatient treatment avoids radical disruption of whatever degree of normalcy clients have been able to maintain despite their illness. Fees are generally on a sliding scale, pegged to income, with Medicaid payment usually accepted. Such programs are cost-effective to city, county and state institutions because outpatient acupuncture treatment is inexpensive. Hospitalization can often be avoided, or if not avoided, curtailed. Treatment of pregnant cocaine users means more babies carried to term and of good birth-weight, thus not requiring intensive-care hospitalization.

The originator of public-health addiction treatment using acupuncture is Lincoln Detox, as many still refer to it (officially, its name is Acupuncture Clinic, Substance Abuse Division, Lincoln Medical and Mental Health Center). The clinic occupies a low, gray-painted brick building on a dead-end street in the Mott Haven section of New York's South Bronx.

Ten years ago Lincoln Detox presented an astounding sight to a first-time visitor familiar with the rowdy, hostile behavior prevailing at an ordinary neighborhood methadone clinic.

This was the scene:

Clients at Lincoln Detox waited their turns calmly outside the treatment room. Newcomers' intake paperwork was quickly done. In the large, bright treatment room forty-nine high-backed padded chairs lined the walls and formed short rows where space permitted. People—primarily poor, Hispanic, and black, from teenagers on up—sat with five long needles dangling from each ear. Some also had needles in their hands, arms, legs and feet. Six cubicles provided privacy for treatments which required that needles be placed in the torso. The six counselor-acupuncturists and three MD/acupuncturists tended their paperwork at a couple of long tables in full view of clients.

People sat as long as they needed to collect themselves once the needles were removed. Some clients got up, removed their own needles, dropped them into the alcohol-filled plastic used-needle container, and left.

The clinic looked casual but in fact all activity was purposeful. Staffers constantly updated clients' cases and discussed clients' progress. There was none of the icy briskness so often associated with hospitals, where matters urgently important to a patient seem to be settled by people who reside behind closed doors. At Lincoln, clinic workers treated clients in a calm, friendly way.

At that time 300 people a day were treated at Lincoln Detox on a low-budget outpatient basis. Medicaid was arranged for indigent clients, and carfare provided. Although most Lincoln clients lived in poverty, the clinic treated people from a wide economic range, including some who could afford to fly to New York, stay in a hotel and travel to the South Bronx by limousine.

Communal treatment serves several purposes. Clients learn from each other by sharing experiences; they get a feeling for the ethnically diverse staff by watching the interaction with other clients. Also, the group setting allays the anxiety many people feel about treatment.

In a corner of the treatment room, a woman with five needles in each ear and no upper front teeth was willing to talk about her experience.

"I have a problem with alcohol," she said. "I needed a program or my children would be taken away." Three of her five children lived with her. "I never took drugs, but that's the only needles I'm scared of."

She had trouble finding a program. She went to one, but was "dry"—that is, she had not recently had a drink—and they wouldn't take her.

"I said, 'You mean, I gotta be drunk 'fore you'll sign me into the alcohol program?'."

When she came to Lincoln, a counselor asked if she had an alcohol problem. She replied that she didn't have a problem; she just liked drinking. She told the counselor that "they" were going to take her children away. "See, I was denying it," the woman said "which really shows you got a problem." For three years she had been coming for daily treatment. During that time she was able to retain custody of her children.

At that time fees ranged from $7 to $28 per treatment, but any annual figure reached by multiplying this woman's treatment by the number of visits would be meaningless in terms of the complexity of health-care finance. Her outpatient treatment was obviously cheaper than the sporadic hospitalizations that are so common in an alcoholic's history. Outpatient treatment made it possible for her to keep her children, a great dollar-saving over what the foster care bill would have been. The social benefit was incalculable.

One patient said of Lincoln, where he went for immune-system treatment, "The whole world is there. You sit and have the relaxing needles first, in the ears, and look around, and there are heroin junkies, and lawyers with briefcases, and Upper East Side ladies, and typists—the whole world. It's an extraordinary sensation to have acupuncture with people from every walk of life."

Two men were at Lincoln on a Saturday morning. One of them spoke as an MD/acupuncturist inserted the last of thirteen needles in his partner, whose face bore grape-purple blotches.

"I'm getting treatment for my immune system, although I don't have anything," said Jake, who started coming to Lincoln Detox mainly to encourage his lover. Quietly, he described his friend's steady improvement in general health over the past six months. Jake had also come to recognize other clients and observe their improvement.

Several staff members spoke about their work. Ana Oliveira, born in Brazil, began working and training here in 1981 while studying for her Master's degree in Medical Anthropology. In 1983 she was hired by King's County Hospital in Brooklyn to set up their acupuncture program; in 1984 she joined the Lincoln staff.✦

✦Some of these staff people later moved on to other jobs in the substance-abuse field. José Aponte, who worked at Lincoln Hospital for nearly twenty years until his death in 1991, treated tens of thousands of people in the South Bronx. Acupuncture masters from many other countries admired and respected his skill.

Oliveira treated clients with acupuncture, carried a caseload of clients whom she counseled regularly, and assisted Lahary Pittman—acupuncturist, counselor, and head coordinator—in managing clinic activities.

José Aponte, acupuncturist, was one of the founders of Lincoln Detox. He said that at first he didn't think much about acupuncture, but gradually took an interest. Acupuncture, he said, was hard to learn.

Kamau Kokayi, MD, took a year off from Yale Medical School to learn acupuncture in a work-study program. His thesis project was to explain acupuncture in terms of Western science.

Acupuncturist and counselor Wendy Cintron said, "I was one of the first clients to try acupuncture. At that time it was electroacupuncture. I really felt good about it. It relaxed me: it helped me through my detox. Once I was detoxed, I wanted to work as a counselor. I wanted to become part of the program, because I felt it helped me. So I volunteered for three years, and then I was hired."

In 1988, the New York City Council heard testimony which confirmed Lincoln's assertion that more than 60 percent of substance abuse clients are retained in acupuncture treatment—a much higher figure than any other form of outpatient drug-free treatment. As the *Harvard Health Letter* stated, Lincoln's 60 percent is "an astonishing rate, given that most are not seeking rehabilitation on their own but rather have been ordered to participate by a judge." Even clients who entered addiction treatment only because the courts ordered it continue their acupuncture treatment after attendance is no longer legally required.

It did not happen overnight . . .

2

DRUG ADDICTION IN THE US: A BRIEF HISTORY

While the use of acupuncture to alleviate addiction is new, the basic idea that addiction is an illness to be treated rather than a crime to be punished is not at all a recent development. In fact, addiction was not widely regarded as a crime in the United States until well into the twentieth century, and drug addiction in the United States did not become a social problem and growth industry until the 1920s. Before the 1830s addicts—most of whom used opium—were not an identifiable population. They either maintained their habits or sought help from local doctors. Morphine, derived from opium and superbly powerful against acute pain, at one time was used as a remedy for opium addiction. As the history of drug abuse treatment in this country shows, while it may seem logical to use one drug against another, it doesn't necessarily work.

During the Civil War morphine was not only given for combat injuries, but also dispensed liberally to cure dysentery among the troops. A severe social problem of the post-Civil War era was widespread morphine addiction, commonly known as "Soldiers' Disease." Heroin, synthesized from morphine, was initially considered nonaddictive, and given to cure morphine addiction. But heroin in the body quickly turns back into morphine; therefore heroin proved every bit as addictive as the drug whose abuse it was intended to cure. Drug abuse has always been medication carried to the extreme.

The hypodermic syringe, invented by a French doctor in 1853, provided a new way to put medication into the body. The last third of the 19th century saw growing morphine use—both by injection and as an ingredient in many newly popular patent medicines. Other patent medicines contained cocaine. Opiates were ingredients in many over-the-counter products at the local drugstore. Heroin tablets, for instance, were sold as cough medication. Street dealing as the retail outlet of major black-market drug businesses did not yet exist.

In 1909 the government banned importation of opium except for medicinal purposes. Heroin, manufactured by Bayer & Bayer in Germany, continued to be imported and sold directly to American consumers until 1915, when the Harrison Narcotics Act of 1914 went into effect.

Drafted as revenue-producing legislation, the Harrison Act included provisions which made possible the eventual stifling of physician-supervised addiction treatment. The Act regulated commercial aspects of legitimate narcotics transaction, formed the basis for subsequent narcotics control legislation and became the tool of political trends and economic interests.

The Harrison Act obliged anyone in any way involved in the business of importing, manufacturing, dispensing, distributing or even giving away coca leaves or opium and its derivatives, to register with the district internal revenue collector, and to pay a special occupation tax.

Doctors, dentists and veterinarians had to be prepared to show records of narcotics prescriptions for the preceding three-month period whenever requested by an authorized internal revenue employee. Failure to comply with Harrison Act requirements was initially punishable by a fine of up to $2,000 and/or up to five years in prison.

Ironically, this law, which was designed to increase federal revenues by taxing opiates and cocaine, resulted in diminishing legitimate drug-importing commerce, thus making the smuggling of such drugs highly profitable. Allowing the Treasury Department, rather than the Public Health Service, to supervise medical use of narcotics and cocaine laid the groundwork for a long-running contest. The Harrison Act became entangled in the growing dispute between those who saw addicts as patients, and those who— sometimes for self-serving political goals—labeled them criminals.

After 1914, private drug-treatment clinics and individual doctors continued to treat patients according to various theories, most commonly by giving ever-smaller doses of the addict's chosen drug. Although increasingly strict enforcement of the Harrison Act did stop a relatively few unethical doctors from writing multiple drug prescriptions for profit, it also had a chilling effect on sincere physicians working in addiction treatment. It became professionally disastrous for doctors to operate private clinics, as they became easy targets for political witch-hunters on the campaign trail. Consequently, starting in 1919, a number of cities throughout the country organized public narcotics clinics. Tension continued between these outpatient clinics and the federal government because the federal view was that detoxification should take place inside an institution, and that abstinence must be enforced. Maintenance or tapering off were anathema. The work of small clinics was disrupted by federal agents' frequent demands to inspect paperwork. Although local governments had established these clinics, federal officials harassed them so zealously that by 1923 they had all closed down.

Drug prices rose, and most addicts turned to an illicit market whose merchants made extraordinary profits on a cheap commodity.

Federal hospitals treating addicts were established at Lexington, Kentucky in 1935, and Fort Worth, Texas in 1938. Part hospital and part prison, these hybrid institutions were

staffed by the U.S. Public Health Service and accepted crimi-
nally charged addicts for compulsory residential treatment.
Other addicts could commit themselves voluntarily for
detoxification. Some people checked themselves into Lexington intending to clean up for good. Others used a voluntary stay at Lexington, which they could quit at will, to
reduce their tolerance enough to be able to get high on
smaller doses when they came out. Eventually studies
showed that 90 percent of the population treated at Lexington relapsed. In 1971, Fort Worth, which still has special
programs for drug and alcohol treatment, was turned over
to the Bureau of Prisons. In 1974, the Bureau took over
Lexington as well—but not its Addiction Research Unit.

Civilians' drug sources dried up temporarily during
World War II, but after the war ended drug use increased.
Yet there was no change in addiction-treatment policy. From
1923 to 1965 there were no public outpatient clinics. For
most addicts, rehabilitation consisted of detoxification by
going "cold turkey" when arrested.

In 1958, when there were no legitimate sources of treatment for addicted Americans except Lexington and Fort
Worth, Synanon, a private therapeutic community of addicts living together in a drug-free environment, was established. At Synanon you had to detox without chemical assistance, but you had the company and support of other
residents. After detoxification and a trial period, new members passed through various phases of assigned work and
increased responsibility.

Other residential therapeutic communities, based more
or less on the Synanon format, appeared in the 1960s, notably Daytop Village, Odyssey House and Phoenix House.
Therapeutic communities were structured like old-fashioned—indeed, Old-Testament—patriarchal families. An
article of faith was the confrontational group therapy session, something like Marine boot camp without the physi-
cal-fitness opportunities.

Youth was a major target of most domestic marketing strategies in the 1960s and 1970s. The drug market was no exception and the treatment market followed suit, which may account for the stern-parent aspect of many therapeutic communities.

However, these drug-free therapeutic communities (which from time to time did not live up to the label), could not possibly take on everyone who needed help kicking addictions.

Methadone, a synthetic morphine-like painkiller originally called dolophine, was developed in Germany during World War II. Like natural opiates, it was used as a cough medicine and to treat severe visceral pain. Shortly after World War II, the federal prison-hospitals began using methadone to detoxify addicts. But methadone didn't stay within the confines of the Public Health Service: people in the drug life soon adopted it to taper off on their own, to ease withdrawal or to get a high—albeit a lesser one—when heroin was hard to find.

The Federal Bureau of Narcotics was established in 1930, and, like the FBI, was for decades the personal fiefdom of a politically savvy commissioner, Harry J. Anslinger. In the early 1960s the narcotics bureau still dominated the care of drug addicts. For nearly forty years the territory might as well have been posted "Doctors Keep Out," except for the Public Health Service. Only a small percentage of young doctors did a PHS stint at Lexington or Fort Worth. With no firsthand clinical experience available to civilian doctors, and with diminishing research possibilities, a scientific medical approach to drug addiction was seriously impeded for forty years.

In 1963, at New York City's Rockefeller Institute, Dr. Vincent Dole and Dr. Marie Nyswander began to investigate drug-use maintenance. They studied addict volunteers at the institute's fifty-bed research hospital. Dole's previous research in metabolism inclined him to think that long-term opiate addicts underwent permanent metabolic changes and thus would always require medication. On this assumption it seemed sensible to stabilize addicts on small, regular doses of a drug that would keep them comfortable and eliminate the need to spend most of their time stealing or hustling to support a habit.

Dr. Nyswander began working with drug addicts in 1945 during her Public Health Service assignment to Lexington. This experience made her think there must be a better way to rehabilitate addicted people. Before her association with Dr. Dole, she had for several years treated addicts at a Manhattan storefront office on East 103rd Street. A trained psychiatrist familiar with urban street life, she shared Dole's opinion that addiction was a disease, not a psychological aberration. Their approach to addicts in the clinical trials at Rockefeller University, and in Manhattan General Hospital and other treatment centers they supervised,was based on their belief that most addicts had a medical problem in addition to multiple social problems, and that human relations were central to rehabilitation.

Dole and Nyswander soon learned they could not stabilize their patients on morphine or heroin, because effects last only about four hours, and because tolerance—the need for increased dosages to prevent withdrawal symptoms—developed. But patients who were given methadone—one of various opiate-like drugs used in the initial study—showed very different responses. They were comfortable for much longer periods, as a dose could prevent withdrawal for twenty-four hours. They did not develop tolerance and they were able to undertake and complete tasks and projects unrelated to drug use.

Even before Dole and Nyswander published an article on their clinical trials of methadone maintenance in the *Journal of the American Medical Association,* some public-health officials welcomed the prospect of setting up addiction-treatment centers based on stabilizing addicts with a reliable legal drug. Within five years a specific residential methadone-detoxification treatment plan, in most cases followed by outpatient methadone maintenance, grew from a radical concept to an official policy. In January 1970, then-Governor Nelson Rockefeller allocated additional funding for the New York State methadone program.

Methadone *maintenance* made outpatient treatment possible, and was politically favored as a cure for addicts' antisocial behavior, even though it rarely cured addiction.

From 1965 onward, methadone treatment had increasing government approval. Government sanction also spawned a gold rush of new methadone programs. These bypassed Dole and Nyswander's original social and therapeutic approach, and instead involved simply handing out methadone and expecting the medication to carry the entire weight of treatment, rehabilitation, and aftercare. Some medical papers questioned pro-methadone maintenance data, and also questioned results of tests that showed methadone was not physically harmful. Poorly designed programs undermined the entire concept.

Long-term experience suggests that methadone was always more popular with social service agencies than with clients. Methadone's side effects, even when the drug is used in an authorized maintenance program, are strikingly similar to those of heroin. These include decreased sex drive, decreased potency, and constipation. Also, methadone is addictive. People who have taken methadone say it's harder to kick than heroin. Its withdrawal symptoms are just as miserable as heroin's. These can include a pounding heart, wheezing cough, shaking, cold sweats, stomach cramps, dilated pupils, excess saliva and thus a constant need to swallow, anxiety, tension, aching bones and a general sense of dread. Infants born affected by methadone suffer a very painful withdrawal period.

Ex-offenders who went to prison with drug habits have reported that cold turkey, even when nasty, is preferable to methadone detox—and to methadone maintenance. "It makes your bones ache," they say; and "your teeth hurt all the time"; and "it's harder to get off methadone than to get off heroin, anytime."

Time and events eroded the early promise of methadone maintenance. Many black and Hispanic urban community activists were saying methadone treatment was nothing but the government's way to cut down street crime without concern for addicted people's health. Why exchange one habit for another, they argued, even if the new drug didn't cost you anything? The more politically militant also insisted that enrolling in a methadone program subjected a person to government blackmail: you could be told that if you didn't pass on to authorities any radical-politics gossip from the neighborhood, you might not get your dose.

One observer of methadone treatment summed it up by commenting, "Methadone was a substitute for what was happening before that, which was nothing. It helped some people, but there were a lot of problems involved with it, because of the limits and standards."

Methadone treatment was the country's only legal medication-detox regimen, yet having achieved hard-won official sanction it proved to be just another step in the erratic record of coping with addicted people in the United States.

3

ACUPUNCTURE: HOW IT WORKS

Evidence that acupuncture could effectively treat substance abuse emerged from a chance discovery in Hong Kong, in 1972. Dr. Hsiang-Lai Wen reported that a fifty-year-old man with a five-year opium habit was admitted to the Kwong Wah Hospital's neurosurgical unit. The man's addiction became evident when he showed signs of withdrawal. To relieve his addiction he agreed to an operation on the nerves in his brain (cingulumotomy), and to be prepared for surgery with the help of acupuncture instead of chemical anesthesia. Needles were inserted at hand, arm and ear points and attached by wires to a machine providing an electrical charge. After a while the patient told the doctors that his withdrawal symptoms had disappeared. The operation was canceled, but the patient remained in the hospital. Later, when withdrawal pangs recurred, he was treated again with acupuncture, and the symptoms again disappeared after about half an hour. Two other opium addicts were treated the following day by the same method, with the same results.

Dr. Wen and his colleague, Dr. S. Y. C. Cheung, subsequently treated forty other heroin and opium addicts with acupuncture, and reported the results in the *Asian Journal of Medicine* in 1973. The same year, the *New York Times* ran an article on electropotentiated ear acupuncture as administered to opiate addicts at Kwong Wah Hospital under the protocol designed by Wen, who said, "We don't claim it's a cure for drug addiction. If we can treat withdrawal symptoms, make a patient more comfortable, and alleviate their suffering, then we have achieved something. Our treatment is not the complete answer to the drug problem." A related *Times* item noted that New York City's Health Commissioner Joseph Cimino knew that acupuncture had been suggested as a possible aid to drug detoxification, but there was no scientific data on it in the United States.

With drug addiction already a multinational problem, the Kwong Wah work drew attention to the use of acupuncture in addiction treatment. In the following years the idea spread at international drug-abuse conferences. Acupuncture was acceptable to patients; it was simple and cheap; it eliminated the need for pharmaceuticals and resulted in shorter hospitalization. Acupuncture-assisted detoxification opened the possibility of rehabilitation treatment on an outpatient basis, which would mean a great cost-saving over inpatient care.

Some explanation of acupuncture is needed to understand why it proved effective against withdrawal symptoms in those Hong Kong addict-patients.

Chinese traditional medicine holds that vital energy, called *qi* (pronounced "chee") circulates throughout the body as does blood. (The concept that blood *and* vitality circulate in a closed system existed in China as early as 200 B.C.E.). Qi moves along pathways called meridians. Of the body's fourteen major meridians: twelve are "paired", that is, they are mirrored on the right and left sides; the other two meridians are single, running up the front and back midline and over the head. Meridians are named after organ systems: Lung, Large Intestine, Stomach, Spleen, Heart, Small Intestine, Urinary Bladder, Kidney, Pericardium, Triple Burner, Gall Bladder, Liver, Conception Vessel and Governing Vessel. Meridians and related organ systems are thought of not only as anatomical entities, but also as physiological functions.

Chinese medical literature assigns each acupuncture point a name that usually suggests either that point's use, its location on the body or its relation to energy flow. In Western acupuncture practice, most points are identified by their location on the meridian. For example, the Chinese name of leg point Tsu San Li means "walk three miles"; in English it is Stomach 36. Western practitioners identify a small category of points not located on meridians with the prefix EM (Extra Meridian). Some acupuncturists favor an international numerical system with a standard number for each point, because the present identification is complicated by language differences. For instance, a Lung point on the thumb is LU 11 to American practitioners but it is P 11 to French ones, as the French word for "lung" is *poumon*.

Early Chinese physicians used auricular acupuncture— treating patients by placing needles at specific points in the external ear. Some ear points have names indicating that they exist only on the ear. But Heart 7, at the wrist, and a point in the upper ear both have the same name, Shen Men—meaning "Spirit Gate"—written with the same Chinese characters. English-speakers commonly say "Ear Shen Men" to distinguish it from the other point.

Renewed interest in auricular acupuncture emerged in China and France almost simultaneously in the 1950s.

One modern Chinese ear-acupuncture map identifies 136 points with indications for treatment of glands, joints, nerves and organs, as well as conditions like asthma, constipation, hepatitis and hypertension. For example, an ear point just inside the rim, about halfway between the apex of the ear and the lobe, is for a shoulder-joint problem. A hunger-control point lies three-quarters of the way between the apex of the tragus and its lower end, halfway between the edge of the tragus and the jawbone.

Paul Nogier, a French doctor, elaborated a system also based on connections between organs and ear points, but using anatomical landmarks slightly different from those used by the Chinese. Nogier demonstrated that ear points are detectable when related systems are dysfunctional.

Yoshiaki Omura, MD, who is also a physicist, experienced acupuncturist and researcher, was originally skeptical of Nogier's diagnostic use of ear points. But in his textbook, *Acupuncture Medicine,* he writes: "Without any prior knowledge of the histories of these volunteer subjects, about 55 per cent of the diseases they had or had previously had were accurately diagnosed through this method."

The effects of ear acupuncture have been explained in various ways. Classic analysis holds that subsidiary connections of meridians pass through the ear. Some contemporary experts say that ear points are related to organs *not* via meridians, but through the central nervous system. Another way to consider ear acupuncture is as a tributary of the larger acupuncture river.

Acupuncture theory says that blocked energy causes imbalance. Disease is an imbalance among parts of the body; an imbalance in the system and an imbalance in the transition from one state of being to another (*yin/yang*). No absolute balance exists in living things, which are always in a state of change, but there is dynamic equilibrium. The body, mind and emotions continually interact, and diagnosis must take account of these interactions.

Standard diagnosis begins with four steps: observation; smelling and listening; questioning the patient and palpating. The latter includes pulse-taking. (In Western medicine, a complete physical examination includes four similar steps: inspection, palpation, percussion—tapping to discern resonance in a part of the body—and auscultation—listening to body sounds, either directly, with the ear, or indirectly, by stethoscope.)

Over the centuries Chinese medicine defined an extensive list of pulse qualities. They include many nuances of the familiar Western values of rate, rhythm, volume and strength. The traditional Chinese way to read pulses is to press the radial arteries of the patient's left and right wrists at three different locations, varying the pressure to read pulses at high, medium and low levels. An experienced acupuncturist can discern a very complex physiological picture by pulse-taking used as a check against other diagnostic information. Acupuncture and pulse-taking allow continuous immediate examination of the patient's reactions.

Another stage of diagnosis identifies and classifies the combinations of signs and symptoms the patient is presenting. For example, one type of headache must be differentiated from other types with different origins.

Chinese medicine diagnoses the dominant cause of the patient's complaint according to external and internal factors and habitual activities. External factors are wind, cold, heat, dampness, dryness and fire. Internal factors are emotions, such as fear, anger, worry and sadness. Habitual activities include eating, drinking, work and sexual activity. Miscellaneous factors include trauma, parasites, internal bleeding and embolism. Each factor in turn is further assessed to form a detailed picture of the patient's condition, composed of the patient's individual pattern of symptoms.

Because Chinese medicine uses methods different from those of Western medicine to activate the same biological system, describing and validating acupuncture according to Western science is a complex task. In the United States the job has been further complicated by a mistrust of empirical medicine, which is based on experience and observation, rather than on testing of hypotheses to form a theory. In this context, however, it is useful to note that for over seventy years medical doctors used at least one medication—aspirin—empirically, without understanding its mechanism, just because it worked. Not until 1971 was there a thorough scientific explanation for *how* aspirin relieves pain.

Studies in Australia, China, France, Germany, Italy, Japan, Russia, Scandinavia and the United States have produced partial analyses of how acupuncture works but to date there is no universally accepted theory.

Laboratory experiments at the single-cell level have demonstrated acupuncture's mechanism; high-tech photography has examined and tracked how the body responds to acupuncture; findings in other fields of inquiry have suggested still further clues. Formal studies of people receiving acupuncture have confirmed anecdotal clinical data. Mainstream English-language peer-reviewed journals such as *Brain Research, European Journal of Neuroscience, Experimental Neurology, Lancet* and *Nature,* have joined the worldwide scientific press in publishing acupuncture-research articles.

Much Western acupuncture research in the 1970s focused on pain. The "gate theory" held that acupuncture blocks the traffic of pain messages—six "pain lines" occupy the spinal cord—to the brain. The "endorphin theory" suggested that acupuncture releases endogenous morphine-like substances into the central nervous system—substances whose narcotic effects alleviate pain.

Bruce Pomerantz, MD, a neurophysiologist and prominent acupuncture researcher who has worked both in the United States and Canada, testified before the Food and Drug administration (FDA) in 1991. Because of his research background and his extensive study of endorphins, Pomerantz's concluding remarks are particularly striking. "I do not think it is all endorphins: *originally we thought it was* [emphasis added] . . . There is a lot more to acupuncture than endorphins . . . There are many things going on here when you insert a needle."

By anatomizing acupuncture, laboratory research into the mechanism of acupuncture attempts to see what those "many things" are.

In 1958, Chinese scientists dissected 324 points, and found nerve formations in all of them. Other experts say that 15 percent of acupuncture points have no relationship to nerves.

Experiments on anesthetized cats observed single-cell response to touch and pain, and the modification of pain response by acupuncture.

Electroacupuncture experiments on rabbits, at Shanghai Medical University's Institute of Acupuncture Research, show that the hormone noradrenaline decreased—and the pain threshold increased—in rabbits during acupuncture stimulation. In other experiments, carotid arteries of two rabbits were linked by plastic tubing to demonstrate cross-circulation of acupuncture analgesia. When the donor rabbit exhibited a higher pain threshold after acupuncture, so did the recipient rabbit. A mechanically similar experiment connected rabbits so that they shared spinal fluid. In this instance also, acupuncture analgesia was shown to travel from the donor rabbit to the recipient.

For several years scientists at Beijing Medical College trying to explain precisely the mechanism of acupuncture analgesia have been investigating the different types of substances that acupuncture releases in laboratory animals, and exploring how these substances determine which rabbits and rats experience analgesia with acupuncture and/or electroacupuncture, and which ones don't.

Another view of acupuncture has emerged by means of thermography, a photographic process which reveals temperature variations in the body. Western investigators showed in a sequence of thermographic color pictures that acupuncture at a hand point between the thumb and the first metacarpal, commonly used to induce analgesia, increases the temperature of the hand. This thermographic demonstration is consistent with clinical observation reported by a Shanghai researcher who said that when acupuncture is used for analgesia, increased skin temperature at palm and finger shows that pain suppression is taking place.

Investigation of meridians by radioactive tracers was undertaken by a French medical team whose report was published in 1985. A camera tracked the movement of ra-

dioactive isotopes injected at acupuncture points. The resulting photographs showed that isotopes traveled along
pathways which matched classical Chinese acupuncture
meridians, pathways which differed from the courses of
lymphatic vessels, blood vessels and nerves.

The concept of *qi*, integral to acupuncture, troubles
Western medical science because *qi* cannot be weighed,
measured or examined by even the most sophisticated mi-
croscope. Does *qi* relate to what Western science knows as
the low-grade electrical current produced by the human
body? Dr. Bjorn Nordenström, former head of diagnostic
radiology at Stockholm's Karolinska Institute and 1985 chairman of Karolinska's Nobel Assembly, published a theory of
biologically closed electrical circuits functioning as an additional circulatory system which regulates chemical and
physical processes. Nordenström was *not* investigating acupuncture, but his work suggests that bio-electromagnetism
could account for acupuncture's effects. However, without
rigorous proof, experts caution against equating *qi* with
bioelectricity. *Qi* remains undefined in Western scientific
terms. It is easier to record acupuncture's effects than to
explain how it produces these effects.

Acupuncture affects nerves, muscles, and hormones, and
has been shown to release cortisone, gonadotrophins, and
thyroxin, among other hormones. An acupuncture needle
in the skin produces an electromagnetic field, which promotes bone- and tissue-healing. Acupuncture at a hand point
has been shown to increase white blood cells, stimulating
the immune system. Acupuncture has a balancing effect on
the autonomic and neurotransmitter systems. It stimulates
liver function, circulation, and waste elimination. Some
experts say that Shen Men, an ear point used in addiction
treatment, affects the hypothalamus, a part of the brain
very close to the pituitary gland which strongly influences
metabolism.

Along with effects which may be objectively recorded,
patients who benefit from acupuncture often say, "I don't
know if it was the acupuncture, I just feel better. Nothing
special happened. Maybe I feel better because my supervi-

sor finally got off my back." Response to acupuncture feels natural and spontaneous.

Whatever the means by which acupuncture affects physiology, enough clinical documentation of ear-acupuncture addiction treatment has accumulated to show that it alleviates withdrawal symptoms, reduces cravings and calms the emotions.

Thousands of chemically dependent patients have been treated and their cases recorded, but clinical histories are less persuasive evidence than studies designed for publication in scientific journals. In the latter, work must be explained so that others can replicate the results by following exactly the same procedures.

Milton Bullock, MD and Patricia Culliton, L.Ac. conducted a landmark pilot study of this type under the aegis of the Chemical Health Division, Hennepin County, Minnesota. Even with a physician on the team—an MD's participation lends Western scientific respectability to acupuncture—developing the clinical research design, performing the study, writing it up and submitting it for publication was a long process. This pilot study, titled "Acupuncture Treatment of Alcoholic Recidivism," appeared in the May/June 1987 issue of *Alcoholism,* the journal of the American Medical Society on Alcoholism. The fifty-four patients studied were unemployed male chronic alcoholics, each of whom had at least twenty admissions to the Hennepin County Detox Center, and no record of successful treatment. Half the patients received standard acupuncture treatment for detox; the others were treated at ear and wrist points not specifically indicated for detox.

Patients were referred as volunteers for the study after three to five days in the detox center. In Phase One, patients received daily acupuncture for five days. In Phase Two, they had treatment three times a week for four weeks and in Phase Three, treatment twice weekly for forty-five days. Thirty-seven percent of the treatment group completed all three phases, but only about 7 percent of the control group did so. This confirmed other centers' clinical observations about acupuncture's power to retain clients in treatment.

Drinking episodes for both groups were about the same in Phase One. Data on Phases Two and Three show many more drinking episodes and detox admissions for the control group than for the treatment group.

On the question of client retention, as well as effectiveness of acupuncture in treating chemical dependency, this closely supervised research supported what clinicians had been seeing since 1974.

4

LINCOLN DETOX, RADICAL SOLUTION

The method of chemical-dependency acupuncture now used on a large scale in U.S. public health settings, and in other countries, evolved at a clinic founded at Lincoln Hospital in New York City. Formally known as the Acupuncture Clinic, Substance Abuse Division of the Department of Psychiatry of Lincoln Hospital, it is still often called by its old name, Lincoln Detox. The original clinic was established as an improvised response to community needs in November 1970. It used methadone to detoxify heroin addicts. Acupuncture has been integral to the clinical program since 1974. Since then, the clinic has become the paramount national and international developer of practice and theory in applying acupuncture to treatment of chemical dependency.

Community self-help was the foundation of Lincoln Detox, where a small professional medical staff worked with large numbers of neighborhood volunteer staffers— among them many former chemical-dependency patients— to treat addicted people. From the outset, addicts themselves were consulted and the work-style was not hierarchical but collective.

The Lincoln program was shaped by the historical context in which it developed, the turbulent period of community activism and radical militancy that characterized the late 1960s and early 1970s. Residents of New York's medically underserved areas in Brooklyn, northern Manhattan and the South Bronx politicized health-care delivery. The central demand was for quality health care for poor people who, in these neighborhoods, were mainly Hispanic and black.

The most compelling health issue, the one which prompted the most municipal and state government discussion and attracted endless press coverage, was drug-abuse treatment. In 1970 a patient might have had to wait as long as a year to enter any type of program in New York City, the center of U.S. heroin addiction. Rising expectations caused friction: people in areas most subject to drug abuse knew that programs existed, and resented the fact that there were too few to satisfy growing demands. A January 1970 *New York Times* editorial titled "No One Answer to Drugs" addressed "the basic need to attack the roots of the drug-abuse problem, which are entwined with the roots of other social problems: housing, education, health care, jobs, family instability, the whole ugly knot of problems which affect so many inner-city residents adversely." This excerpt is still applicable.

In areas where drug abuse flourished and affected ever-younger people, residents used civil rights- and anti-war-movement tactics to claim satisfaction from an unresponsive municipal health-care system. The year 1970 was notable for civil disruption. Sit-ins and demonstrations were commonplace. Students sat in demanding university curriculum changes; mothers picketed and invaded City Hall demanding bus passes for schoolchildren. As a political tactic the sit-in let otherwise powerless people force an issue, rather than allowing it to drift away on an ocean of vague assurances where the buck never stopped. A Manhattan church was the site of an eight-hour sit-in by a group demanding space for an addiction rehabilitation center. In upper Manhattan the Community Psychiatry Unit of St. Luke's Hospital experienced a four-day sit-in by Mothers Against Addiction and members of a street academy called ABLE, who demanded treatment facilities for heroin addicts younger than eighteen. (The City Medical Examiner's Office statistics showed that over 25 percent of those who died from heroin overdoses were between twelve and nineteen.) Community groups orchestrated a demonstration at Harlem Hospital in northern Manhattan, where 200 drug addicts sat in, demanding addiction treatment. The Young Lords and the Health Revolutionary Unity Movement organized a takeover of Lincoln Hospital, then located on 141st Street, near Southern Boulevard, resulting in a tumultuous period of community demands, ousters, doctors' walkouts and abrupt staff changes.

In November, several groups joined together as United Bronx Drug Fighters and demanded that a drug-detoxification center be established immediately at Lincoln Hospital. The hospital had no drug treatment program, although severely ill addicts who turned up in its emergency room were hospitalized.

This was the climate in which Michael O. Smith, MD, after a one-year internship at Harlem Hospital, began a three-year community psychiatry residency at Lincoln Hospital. In the summer of 1970 he was in his second residency year, working at a therapeutic community he described as "loosely sponsored by the hospital," when the Lincoln Hospital takeover occurred.

Recalling the events of 1970, Smith said, "There were a number of other issues regarding the hospital takeovers, but basically what happened was that the Lincoln Detox program grew out of that. Lincoln Detox program started in November 1970, as a suggestion of an ongoing group. We had gotten a lot of doctors at Lincoln to be willing to double up in their dorm rooms so that we could really run a detox unit at Lincoln . . ." [using space in the doctors' residence].

"We had a meeting in community and this one fellow, Butch Ford, had been detoxing people with methadone in his own basement—he was on a maintenance program and would not use all his whole dosage and so he just detoxed people in his own basement. He had quite a few people he'd detoxed. So we called this meeting to run a program, and the patients all volunteered to bring food and come on a certain day, and various other people were going to do leaflets and so on.

"When the day came, at noon we just walked in and took the elevator and went up to the sixth floor. The patients all came, but the people who were going to hand out leaflets and all that didn't do it. Later in the day there was a symbolic arrest of various people in the program. That lasted a few hours.

"Over that weekend there was a discussion with the then chairman of psychiatry, Gabe Koz, and some of us who were involved. And they said, 'Well, Monday morning we're going to do an outpatient methadone detox program.'

"None had ever been done before. There were outpatient *maintenance* programs, but outpatient *detox* means you just give them methadone for ten days and taper the dose.

"There were about 200 people waiting in line the next day. We had a jar of methadone pills on the stage—we had a thousand pills in a jar. And we had virtually no professional staff at all. So we asked people waiting in line if they could help read and write, and do some of the paperwork."

This collective and cooperative work style, combining the knowledge and experience of former patients with the medical skills of the small professional staff, characterized Lincoln Detox from the outset. As the startup work continued, another local volunteer, Vicente "Panama" Alba, who had recently gotten himself clean, became deputy director.

Lincoln Detox workers always had a strong sense of mission to have patients become drug-free, and to stop the drug plague.

"We had a huge volunteer group," Smith said, "and we started in the auditorium of Lincoln Hospital. We were an innovative program from the beginning. We were the only outpatient detox program. And we immediately served a lot of patients in the hospital. Nursing people, a lot of people were very sympathetic, because this was a service-oriented thing."

Because Lincoln Detox was established in response to community action, community people felt they had a stake in running it. Even nonactivists had been saying that black and Hispanic neighborhoods must develop their own institutions, their own cures and their own programs for dealing with the drug blight. Many of Lincoln Detox's volunteer drug counselors also strongly believed that political education was fundamental to rehabilitation. One aspect of political education was to teach clients about the narcotics trade, that the big scores in the drug business were made by people and organizations remote from even the most prosperous street-drug merchant.

From a minority perspective, it made good sense to define drug pushing in black and Hispanic communities as an aspect of racist politics, best countered by encouraging psychosocial awareness, dignity and autonomy. Political education also included social competence: how to deal with the landlord who never fixes the boiler, how to enroll in educational or vocational programs, register to vote, get a copy of your birth certificate, etc. If people coming off drugs could be educated to cherish their own lives, they would consider themselves too valuable to hand over to drug dealers.

Two months into its existence—on January 14, 1971—the New York State Narcotics Addiction Control Commission awarded Lincoln Detox a matching grant of $1,128,388 according to which the city match of state funds could either be in cash or in-kind goods and services. Enough money trickled down through the bureaucratic labyrinth for the program to hire about sixty people. By July, when funds came through, the staff was paid retroactively. Lincoln Detox had relied for eight months on volunteers who performed important nonprofessional tasks.

At the same time, thanks to James Reston's July 1971 front-page article in the *New York Times,* the American public discovered acupuncture. During the next few years, while acupuncture was very much in the news, Lincoln Detox counselors were looking for natural healing methods which could ease patient discomfort during the ten-day methadone detoxification process.

Having completed his three-year psychiatric residency at Lincoln Hospital, Smith began working part-time at Lincoln Detox.

"We started using acupuncture certainly in early 1974, probably even late '73; and I say *we* in that I had very little to do with acupuncture in the beginning. I was working in a storefront outreach program and part-time at the Bronx County Jail."

In this period after President Richard Nixon's visit to China, the press was full of reports about that country. Feature pieces on acupuncture appeared regularly in newspapers and national magazines. By 1973, acupuncture for addiction treatment had become a topic of institutional discussion in this country. Reports of the Kwong Wah hospital work were of special interest to Lincoln Detox personnel.

Smith observed, "In 1974 many of us were discouraged about the use of addictive drugs to treat substance abuse. We turned to natural healing methods, employing at first the drug detoxification protocol of Dr. Wen in Hong Kong."

Much of the pressure for an alternative to methadone came from the clients themselves. One veteran Lincoln Detox staffer recalled, "It was the *clients* that wanted something else besides methadone. We had old methadone users— I'm talking 30, 35, 40 years, which is old in addiction—and they wanted another method of detox, because they didn't like the methadone. They were really dead set on us finding another method for them to detox, and stay clean. That's how we *really* got into acupuncture."

According to Smith, several counselors proposed acupuncture after reading about it in the newspapers. "Two doctors and several counselors tried to dig up some people who would show us. It wasn't too hard, there were various Asian doctors who were interested."

Several acupuncturists came to Lincoln to demonstrate treatment. Smith and others at the clinic were quite surprised that something as seemingly delicate as acupuncture could have an effect on something so powerful as heroin withdrawal symptoms. (This surprise at observing acupuncture's effectiveness is still common, even though by now many Americans have either experienced the treatment or at least are aware of it.)

Eminent acupuncturists and doctors of traditional Chinese medicine donated their time to Lincoln Detox's pioneer program, because it seemed in the public interest. According to Smith, Fung Ngor Wong, MD, was the first person who really helped provide the treatment. Yoshiaki Omura, MD, gave technical instruction and undertook research. Mario Wexu, D.Ac., taught acupuncture for three years at Lincoln Detox.

Based on the methods used at Kwong Wah Hospital to prepare opium-addicted patients for surgery, early acupuncture treatment at Lincoln Detox involved placing one electropotentiated needle at Lung point in the ear—easily locatable in the lower concha. "This gave a reasonably good result with heroin detox," Smith says, "except the effect of treatment did not last very long—only about six hours. For outpatients, and for the economic situation, it became impossible. They had acupuncturists on demand twenty-four hours a day at the Hong Kong hospital."

The Kwong Wah model demonstrated acupuncture's effectiveness in treating addicts. But a less labor-intensive procedure, adapted for outpatient treatment, was obviously needed for an American setting. Today's protocol results from years of modifications developed in clinical work with thousands of patients at Lincoln Detox.

On June 13, 1974, Governor Nelson Rockefeller signed the first New York State law regarding acupuncture. It was restrictive, essentially permitting the investigative use of acupuncture by "qualified practitioners," and leaving it to the State Boards for Medicine and Dentistry to set professional guidelines and standards. The law emphasized compilation of data whose analysis would show how well acupuncture worked. Eventually, under the 1974 law, nonphysician acupuncturists were licensed if they met certain standards and also had ten years' experience in a locality whose licensing regulations were approved by New York's State Board of Education.

At this juncture, Lincoln Detox started using acupuncture with city approval and state enthusiasm. However, establishing acupuncture as a new tool in addiction treatment, and causing the process to flourish, was not an automatic consequence of official acceptance. Smith and his collaborators use cool, analytical and understated terms when recounting Lincoln Detox's acupuncture history in public testimony, presentations to professional groups here and abroad, in journal articles and in press interviews. They describe the work as if it were simple, the way Captain Joshua Slocum wrote of sailing alone around the world aboard a thirty-seven-foot boat. But given the circumstances in which staff and clinic personnel treated patients, it was heroic.

As noted, a coalition of many factions had worked to force establishment of Lincoln Detox; but this collaboration did not result in general agreement on how to operate the clinic.

The Young Lords were a radical Puerto Rican group which for several years had joined other community people and hospital workers in direct actions to force improvement of health care at Lincoln Hospital, and to establish a drug treatment center. The Black Panthers, a militant black group, had also supported the drive for a drug clinic.

In the 1970s radical urban groups often conducted needed programs, such as providing free breakfast or after-school activities for community children. Without claiming the clinic as one of their own programs, the Young Lords visibly ran Lincoln Detox. They did not supplant medical staff, but they did assign non-medical staff to security tasks, and in other ways exerted authority at the clinic. They also taxed clinic workers for the Political Prisoners' Fund—10 percent of their paychecks unless they had more than one child. To a lesser extent, the Panthers were also a continuing presence in the clinic's early existence.

As one veteran clinic worker explained, "The thing that is important to underscore is, without that spirit there wouldn't have been a program. That was why they felt it was right to impose this kind of thing. We look back and say we might not go for that now. But if it wasn't for that kind of forcefulness in saying, 'We stick up for the community,' there wouldn't have been any program."

The clinic's radical genesis flavored its daily routine. A nurse who does chemical-dependency acupuncture in another city hospital recalled working at Lincoln Detox. "I worked at the clinic from the beginning, because they needed a person with a license [to dispense methadone]. I had my year-old daughter with me there; she grew up at Lincoln Detox. There were some others—we called them the Detox Kids."

"When I first came to Lincoln it was 1973," a staff member reminisced, "and we were giving out methadone for detoxification. It was a political program at the time. We had a *lot* of political activists around. We worked in the auditorium at the old Lincoln Hospital nurses' residence.

We would give out methadone on the stage, and the clients would be down on the floor, and there were a lot of revolutionary folks down there.

"Matulu Shakur—he was later on the FBI's 10 Most Wanted list—was the assistant director at that particular time. Zubair was the director when I first came here. They had a lot of political agenda.

"In using the acupuncture, once we got the client clean, they began to *think*. Started asking themselves, 'How come I got no heat or hot water? And my kid can't read? And I'm on welfare but I'm not getting enough money to do so-and-so?'

"So now you got to start doing the talking so they can get back and access the system. The system's not an easy place to be, even if you have a job. So we used to have political education classes. It went over very well with the clients, but not too well with the administration."

Large numbers of patients entered and left the no-frills, outpatient walk-in clinic for morning and afternoon sessions. Disputes and even violence easily carried over from drug-ridden neighborhoods into the clinic. Staff veterans say you never knew what surprises they'd find when they came to work at the old nurses' residence auditorium. One recalled, "We had a man run through there one morning early. He wore the African garb, reached down inside his dashiki and pulled out a machete as big as me, and he went running through the auditorium, chasing somebody! You just stepped to the side—so here we go again!"

Regardless of whatever reckless behavior erupted among clients, and despite differences of political views among the sixty original staff members, Lincoln Detox never shut down. Despite the capricious pressures of neighborhood politics, Lincoln Detox workers persevered, treating 350 patients a day, and providing acupuncture to ease methadone detoxification. A growing proportion of patients relied on acupuncture instead of methadone.

From the beginning there was emphasis on a direct, practical style of working with addicted people. Nancy Smalls, LPN, explained, "We had at least five nurses who worked with us as we were giving out methadone at different hours. Naturally we wore street clothes, because uniforms were very intimidating to this particular clientele." This common-sense approach later provoked misunderstanding at the administrative level.

Other causes of Lincoln Hospital's uneasiness with the clinic were rooted in the social circumstances of Lincoln Detox's origins. Security was an issue: methadone may be distributed only under government license, and supplies must be locked up. As one staffer recalls, "You had a lot of different gangs out there. So you got the tough guys in the neighborhood to be security. The other gangs knew that these guys were there and they stayed away. Not only the people in the street, but a lot of the administration too, didn't want to get involved, because *they* were scared. There was a lot of intimidation."

Intimidation extended to staff meetings, which were conducted according to the participatory-democracy format favored by radical activists. One woman said that during staff meetings the auditorium was locked, and no one was allowed to leave until the issues on the agenda were resolved.

Only a few months after the official launching of acupuncture treatment in mid-1974, terminal violence invaded Lincoln Detox.

The only public account of this disaster appeared in the clinic's newsletter:

PEOPLE'S DOCTOR MURDERED!

On October 29, 1974, at 7:30 A.M. Dr. Richard Taft was found dead in a storage closet in the back of the auditorium of Lincoln Detox. He was one of the doctors who worked in the Lincoln Detox drug program. We, his coworkers, believe that Richie was killed.

Richard was found lying on his side, with his long sleeve shirt and dungaree jacket buttoned at the cuff. An empty syringe was found along with a medical tourniquet and 7 empty glassine bags of the type that street heroin is sold in. However, there were no matches, no cooker or keys to the room. Both doors to the storage closet were found ajar. These doors were always kept locked. Richard's wallet and money were found on his body.

The coroner's office reported finding no needle marks and no heroin in his urine. However heroin was found in his tissues. Richard's body had a large bruise and indentation in the back of the head and scratches on his wrists. The cause of his death has not yet been determined.

The theory that he gave himself a fatal injection is proven false on several counts. Richard was not addicted to heroin or suicidal; if he had given himself an injection, he would not have had time to roll down his sleeves and button them. A fresh needle mark should have been very easily found. Richard was lying in an extremely unnatural position, which raised the possibility that his body had been placed in a container, like the trunk of a car, and then moved.

Two months prior to his death, Richard was shot at by unknown assailants. For the past couple of months Richard had been carrying a weapon for personal protection. As recently as a week prior to his death, he stated to one of our workers that he was in fear of his life and wanted to take a leave of absence.

On the day of his death he was due to meet a high ranking Washington official about the funding of the Lincoln Detox Acupuncture Program. It must also be pointed out that the moment the people from Washington walked into Detox, a telephoned bomb threat was received at the hospital.

These circumstances lead us to believe that

Richard met with some violence prior to his death, that he was shot up with heroin after death or just prior to dying, and that the injection was administered by parties unknown.

The newsletter cited specific threats against Taft, including telephone calls to his home, and concluded, "The most likely explanation of this incident is that Dr. Richard Taft was murdered, by parties unknown in an extremely professional manner, with an obvious attempt to discredit the Lincoln Detox Program."

The newsletter also included a eulogy written by Taft's friends and coworkers. Excerpts give a flavor of Lincoln Detox ambience:

"In Memory of Richard Taft

"Richard Taft, a man, a doctor and above all, a revolutionary. As a man he supported the right and fought the wrong.

"For over four years he served in the South Bronx community. He served for one year as medical doctor in the People's Program, Lincoln Detox. He was instrumental in training paramedics and researching acupuncture as the non-chemical treatment for narcotic withdrawal. It is perhaps this involvement that led to his death.

"He dedicated his life to help people fight their addiction problems with his medical and acupuncture knowledge. It was this dedication that made him continue his work even under the threat of death, even after being shot at. STOP THE DRUG PLAGUE!"

As Smith recalled, "When Richard died I had been doing the statistics and the physicals downstairs while Richard did the treatment upstairs, so there was certainly an *appearance* that Richard was the only person doing treatment. He had in no sense created or invented the acupuncture, but he was following a path and working very hard at it.

"On that day in 1974, we figured that somebody would close the program, but nobody ever did. That's how I became director of the program—the guy who was before me was killed."

5

LINCOLN DETOX, ACUPUNCTURE RESOLUTION

Even as Richard Taft's body was discovered, the auditorium was filling with patients. While police examined the scene, clinic workers carried on. The urgent needs of people on methadone detox had to be served. To retain the clients' confidence, continuity was indispensable.

Although Lincoln Detox was still a methadone program, clinical experience had accumulated to show that acupuncture not only made clients more able to stay off drugs and alcohol but also attracted new program clients.

A persistent problem in drug programs is that clients drop out. Another pitfall is that addicts who clean up notice a whole new series of minor afflictions. (Former heavy tobacco smokers often say, "I stopped smoking because it made me cough, and now I cough more than ever, and my nose runs.") Eliminating drug toxicity from your system is a triumph; having to cope with the physiological responses of a body no longer numbed by drugs is discouraging. Detoxification also brings a revival of sensitivities and emotions which slumbered during the drug-abusing period, so that living clean can involve renewed anguish.

Unlike medication, acupuncture allows change rather than forcing it, while it nourishes and supports both body and emotions. From the earliest use of acupuncture at Lincoln Detox, staffers observed that mandated clients—people directed by court order to attend drug treatment programs—continued acupuncture-based treatment, or returned to it, even when no longer obliged to.

Lincoln Detox was producing notable advances in addiction treatment. However, as is often the case when new ideas are brought to public service, the work itself was the easy part.

From time to time, institutional disputes erupted between Lincoln Hospital and Lincoln Detox. These were inevitable given that Lincoln Detox was the product of a shotgun marriage between the alienated South Bronx community and the hospital. When Lincoln Hospital's new building at 149th Street and Morris Avenue opened in 1976, hope was publicly expressed that new, larger quarters would solve many of the hospital's internal problems, and end its longstanding failure to satisfy community demands for acceptable health care.

Lincoln Detox occupied a clinic area on the new hospital building's first floor. The program also occupied an old former Public Health Station a few blocks away on East 140th Street, where aftercare activities were offered to clients who had completed detox. Acupuncture classes were also held there.

The relationship of Lincoln Detox to Lincoln Hospital, hardly more than détente,was easily upset by complaints and rumors which jeopardized the program's continued existence. At one time, hospital administrators were told that addicts were dispensing methadone and giving acupuncture to other addicts without medical supervision. In fact, the apparent nonmedical personnel were registered nurses (RNs) and licensed practical nurses (LPNs) continuing their practice of wearing street clothes at work. The inaccurate observation and resulting "news" got TV play. Sensational media coverage did not improve clinic-hospital relations.

The good news emerged less dramatically. Outsiders were paying serious attention to Lincoln Detox's use of acupuncture. From the earliest days when acupuncture was demonstrated at the clinic, acupuncturists and professionals in the drug treatment field had been interested in the program. It became important not only to do the work, but also to make public what was learned from this new use of an old therapy.

Members of the Lincoln Detox clinical team testified and made presentations before Congress at the 1976 national hearings on the heroin epidemic; in 1977 they also appeared at the World Congress on Acupuncture in Montreal and in 1978 at the National Drug Abuse Conference in Seattle. In explaining how natural healing methods, including acupuncture, could usefully enhance both drug-free and medication-based programs, they defined Lincoln Detox's central theme: the goal of treatment is to benefit the patient, not to protect institutional turf. As Lincoln Detox's reputation grew in the addiction-treatment community, this focus on the patient eased collaboration with public health, social welfare, and criminal-justice agencies.

Seven months after the Seattle conference, however, when the clinic was treating 200 patients a day, it nearly ceased to function.

In New York City's 1970s antipoverty world, any program benefiting and employing poor minority people became a convenient target for blame when any one of many competing political factions questioned its funding. Accusations of corruption against poverty programs were sometimes accurate, sometimes trumped-up. Inept performance occasionally was the kernel of truth used to justify launching a major exposé. Such scandals often served to divert media attention from trouble brewing in some other fiefdom of New York City's forever-feudal political realm.

Lincoln Detox, while not technically an antipoverty program, was one in spirit. Late in 1978 Mayor Edward Koch's administration reacted to reports that Lincoln Detox was grossly mismanaged. Agencies were called to task for not having monitored the program more closely. The agencies said in self-defense that attempts to control the clinic had been met with threats of violence, and by further threats to close down the entire hospital through picketing and sit-ins. An unidentified member of the Health and Hospitals Corporation (HHC) quoted in the *New York Times* publicly expressed the only common sense: "We find it hard to justify cutting out $100,000 in waste if it means that we lose millions in the event of a retaliatory close-down of Lincoln Hospital."

On the Monday after the 1978 Thanksgiving holiday, a legislator speaking to reporters accused HHC and the State Division of Substance Abuse Services of shielding a mismanaged program. The next evening, under orders from Mayor Koch, HHC's president supervised the program's physical eviction from Lincoln Hospital. In the morning Lincoln Detox workers arrived to see that the police had cordoned off the hospital.

Eyewitnesses recalled the scene. "They locked the door," one man said. "We had to show ID to get into the building. And if we worked for Detox, we weren't allowed in the building."

"They had a *truck* chain! They chained our door together," a woman added, outraged even in retrospect. "We were to be arrested on sight! They took all the records and everything. They thought we were through. They didn't know about this building [the present site of Lincoln Detox on East 140th Street]. So we just came here."

The episode had a characteristically Lincoln Detox outcome—enhancement-by-disaster. The program had virtually phased out methadone in favor of acupuncture; now necessity completed the job. A senior staff member involved in the clinic's dramatic relocation said, "We couldn't bring methadone over here because this building is not good on security. We had to quit giving out methadone. Then we had to really get into acupuncture full-time. We were getting away from methadone, anyway, because it was a drug, and we were against drugs."

The immediate effect was loss of those clients who relied exclusively on methadone, and of others afraid to be associated with a program that was in some kind of trouble. But persistence in bringing acupuncture treatment to clients during a difficult stage in the clinic's life transformed compulsory change into opportunity. Lincoln Detox's reliance on acupuncture established the clinic's unique position in the field of addiction treatment.

Making an end-run around city administration meant that Lincoln Detox was based entirely in the former Public Health Station, where auxiliary services had been offered since the new hospital building opened. Staff people described their workplace. "When we first moved the place was a dump—the conditions that we were working under were real bad. We had to work with umbrellas over our heads!"

"We stuck with it. We stayed in here over a year with no heat, in the cold, and we continued working, giving acupuncture, and thank God for Dr. Smith, 'cause the place would have been *through* if it wasn't for him."

Sometimes Lincoln Detox took the clinic to the people in mobile units. Three addiction counselors remembered those days. "We used to do it in our vehicles on Saturdays and Sundays," says one.

"There was one clinic car here. There was another clinic that would take place at Davoe Park, up by Fordham Road."

"We used to do it by Concourse. They used to come to us on a holiday, Thanksgiving, Christmas. We'd tell 'em, 'We'll be here, and we'll treat you, from a certain time to a certain time.' And we were there."

After the ouster from Lincoln Hospital's building, hospital administration formally designated the clinic the Substance Abuse Division of the Department of Psychiatry. (Around the world, people in the drug-treatment field refer to the clinic as Lincoln Hospital. In the United States the original name persists colloquially: Lincoln Detox.)

Reorganization took place at the 140th Street location. Some clinic workers were reassigned, each to a different hospital. People who believed the acupuncture program should serve political ends, left. Those who remained with the program had felt from the beginning that Lincoln Detox's entire reason for existence was to provide service to addicted people.

The move to 140th Street began a period of regrouping, restaffing and building up the client census, as many patients were lost in the wake of eviction from the Lincoln Hospital building. It was difficult to expand services during those years. Lincoln Hospital's bond with Lincoln Detox continued to be brittle. The 140th Street building did not receive hospital housekeeping services, so clinic staff mopped floors and carried out garbage.

Veteran staffers recall that hospital employees didn't want to work at Lincoln Detox, and they were sometimes assigned to 140th Street when their work at the hospital was unsatisfactory. "But things have changed," a staffer said cheerfully in late 1991. "They've been falling over each other trying to work here now."

The elements which make today's Lincoln Hospital Acupuncture Clinic program so effective were not all identified at once. Through the years, modifications were incorporated into treatment and into the program.

Electrostimulation had been used for about two years when one day the machines broke down. By the time this happened, continuing instruction by professional acupuncturists had given clinicians additional effective points to use with plain needling—for example, Shen Men, in the triangular fossa—along with the electropotentiated Lung point.

As Smith recalls the transition, "We had some needles without electro, but we'd never done it without any." Members of the Lincoln team were parked in a Volkswagen van when a man in extreme distress approached them for treatment. "We're sitting in this hot little truck; you start the machine and the light doesn't go on. It rattles and it's all loose. I thought, well, you can't do this. It won't be strong enough. So we put the needle in, and you try to twirl it, make the effect stronger, with more power."

The prevailing wisdom was that you cured drug abuse with power.

"The more power the better. If the treatment isn't working, turn it on. We all did that; the addicts wanted it, everybody wanted to do that. No one had a clue that you could do it in a different way. The idea that you can gain something by being gentle and simple took a while to be real. In fact a lot of power just gives temporary symptom relief."

While the machine was being repaired, the team's acupuncture skills improved. This was not only a question of achieving greater proficiency by learning more points, but also of adopting the acupunctural concept that less is more, that illness often yields more completely to insinuation than to assault.

Using more precisely located ear points brought improved results without the electropotentiation. In the long run, using plain needles made for a cheaper and more flexible method, an easier-to-learn technique, and a more easily replicated program design.

Following a presentation at the 1977 World Congress of Acupuncture in Montreal, Lincoln Detox was awarded six scholarships for clinicians. The July/September 1979 issue of *The American Journal of Acupuncture* carried a letter from Smith that included these details of a significant stage in the clinic's growth.

Last month we were able to announce the most gratifying accomplishment of the Lincoln Detox Acupuncture Program. Five workers in our program, Walter Bosque, Richard Delaney, Richard Murphy, Mutulu Shakur, and Roxanne Squires, earned the Doctor of Acupuncture (D.Ac.) degree. Dolores Serrano received a level two diploma. These degrees were awarded following a year-long examination period by the Acupuncture Association of Quebec. This association provides a doctoral level training program in acupuncture. . . . During the training period each student spent one month in Montreal as a clinical acupuncturist under supervision. Our teacher, Mario Wexu, spent a number of weeks at Lincoln Detox, providing supervision and personalized instruction. The doctor of acupuncture degree was awarded on a basis of mastery of the entire field of acupuncture.

By 1982 the clinic had clearly defined its detoxification method and treatment plan using acupuncture on drug and alcohol abusers. Protocol details were published in a 1982 issue of *The American Journal of Acupuncture,* in an article by Michael O. Smith, MD, Roxanne Squires, D.Ac., José Aponte, D.Ac., Naomi Rabinowitz, MD, D.Ac. and Regina Bonilla-Rodriguez, S.W. (Most papers produced by Lincoln Detox have multiple bylines.) They were:

❖ ear acupuncture at ear points selected from Shen Men, Sympathetic, Kidney, Liver and Lung
❖ additional points on the hand if the patient was agitated
❖ extra points on ankle and heel for people struggling to overcome addiction to methadone
❖ daily treatment for two to five days for most drugs, except methadone which required up to two months

Drug-program specialists came from other parts of the country and from abroad to observe and to learn to apply the method in their own treatment centers. Lincoln Detox gave on-site training sessions for programs in eight other states. These workshops had three main goals: to demonstrate the usefulness of acupuncture detox to both clinic and client; teach the techniques, uses and limitations of ear-acupuncture treatment; and collaborate with host clinicians in forming an acupuncture component in the local center.

In early 1982 the clinic began also using acupuncture to

help people with immune-related complaints of unknown origin. Later that year the unknown syndrome had an official name: AIDS.

As the message spread that acupuncture was effective in chemical-dependency treatment, demand for training grew. In 1985 a small group of chemical-dependency professionals joined with Smith and senior acupuncturists at Lincoln Detox to form the National Acupuncture Detoxification Association (NADA). NADA's purposes were to establish and maintain a standard for training and certifying a new type of health care worker, the "Acupuncture Detoxification Specialist," someone with a working knowledge of chemical-dependency treatment who is further trained in a specific, limited form of acupuncture. From the outset, NADA literature emphasized that acupuncture for chemical dependency was an *additional* tool to be used in comprehensive rehabilitative programs, and that acupuncture enhances the client's ability to engage in treatment. There was no suggestion that ear acupuncture alone could do the whole job.

In 1985 the crack (smokable cocaine) epidemic began, flooding hospital emergency rooms, overwhelming treatment centers and presenting new treatment challenges. There was no medication for crack analogous to methadone for heroin detox.

Heroin is narcotic, a downer, a depressant. Crack is an upper, a stimulant. Smith wasn't certain how well the points used for heroin and alcohol would work on crack users. Aponte told him he thought most of the clients were already using cocaine. Aponte and Smith spoke with clients in the treatment room, and sure enough, three-quarters of those identified as heroin and alcohol users described how acupuncture also helped reduce their craving for cocaine.

That, says Smith, was a simple discovery which took about three minutes, and came about by consulting the patients. "The discovery came from having a healthy clinic where patients can tell you what to do."

The following year 70 percent of Lincoln Detox's new intakes were crack users, and the patient census increased steadily.

Lincoln Detox's influence expanded, nationally and internationally, while its work continued at a steady pace. By 1986, visitors from thirty-five foreign countries had come to Lincoln Detox. Over 150 alcohol- and drug-treatment center employees had been trained in the Lincoln/NADA protocol. NADA training teams were also invited to distant locations. On-site they would demonstrate acupuncture, train local staff and supervise the process of integrating acupuncture work with the local program. Consultation continued long-distance after the training session.

Lincoln Detox also grew internally, formalizing and expanding services to people with AIDS, to clients referred by criminal justice agencies and to women. Clients, many of whom occupied more than one category, benefitted from the clinic's determination to maintain good working relationships with referring agencies.

Two New York State supervisory agencies had approved acupuncture components, based on the Lincoln model, for existing programs. The Division of Substance Abuse Services (DSAS) had approved an acupuncture training contract for Lincoln to set up five new programs during 1987-1988. Despite this successful record, the New York State Health Department declared on October 2, 1987 that non-physicians must stop administering acupuncture at the clinic.

For fourteen years counselors trained in ear acupuncture had performed most of the clinic's routine detox treatment under medical supervision, or that of licensed acupuncturists. The health department's finding seriously jeopardized the clinic. At the least, 200 clients a day could be prevented from receiving treatment.

This new threat affected the clinic for most of a year, during which a smaller staff worked longer hours, while acupuncture-certified physicians performed all ear-acupuncture treatment for drug and alcohol patients.

Time-consuming political lobbying was the only way to formulate amended state legislation and ensure its sponsorship. To be persuasive at the state level, elected city officials needed to understand the Lincoln program's value.

Smith addressed the New York City Council at the end of June 1988, pointing out that more than 60 percent of substance abuse clients are retained in acupuncture treatment, a much higher figure than that seen in any other form of outpatient drug-free treatment.

Educational lobbying efforts were successful, and on September 1, 1988, Democratic Governor Mario Cuomo signed new legislation, sponsored by Republican State Senator James Donovan, authorizing the training of chemical dependency counselors in detoxification acupuncture under supervision of licensed acupuncturists or doctors. The law made clear that such supervision meant general, on-site clinical supervision, not close, immediate personal supervision. (This 1988 law became section 8216 of the 1991 law on acupuncture.) The Acupuncture Detoxification Training Institute was established, formalizing a process begun twelve years earlier.

Through turbulence and trouble, the Lincoln program refined a method of health care delivery which is essentially peace-inducing.

It is not only the use of acupuncture—in the limited sense of *needling*—that distinguishes addiction treatment at Lincoln Detox from the methods and style of other drug-treatment programs. Program organization is altered because of the use of acupuncture. The essentials are both concrete and intangible.

Chinese medicine views the chemically dependent person as "depleted," as we would say, lacking inner vitality. The acupuncturist notes that such a patient's pulses are generally depressed; other physiological signs indicate suppressed function in certain (yin) organ systems.

Addicted people often exhibit activity described by Chinese words *xu hu*, meaning "empty fire." It's an accurate image of the angry, hustling, frenzied, overbearing behavior common to inner-city addicts. But the strength of Chinese medicine's analysis is that the "empty fire" concept applies equally to all addicts, rich or poor, who engage in restless, unproductive busyness. No matter the socioeconomic group, chemically dependent people dose themselves against fear and dread.

Over time and with experience Lincoln Detox staffers came to appreciate that instead of assaulting the "fire" and trying to douse it, acupuncture nourishes a person's inner emptiness. Acupuncture for detoxification is a simple, non-verbal, repetitive treatment that immediately makes the person feel better and affects him or her profoundly. With daily treatment the patient becomes increasingly calm and clearheaded. As fear and dread subside, so does the busy, flickering, defensive "fire."

Acupuncture's beneficial effects are clear to the person receiving it; in a group setting other clients can also observe these effects. The atmosphere in an acupuncture detoxification clinic is noncompetitive. People sitting in the same room with two-inch needles protruding from their ears are equalized. Nobody is center stage. Acupuncture's calming effect and the sense of clarity and well-being it induces go beyond the individual and pervade the clinic's entire ambience. New clients might behave aggressively or "strut their stuff," but with no payoff of gratifying attention from experienced acupuncture patients, they quickly drop the hostile display.

Clients learn to become responsible by removing their own needles and placing them in a designated container, thus contributing to clinic efficiency. Clients are also responsible for taking home their own "Sleep Mix"—tea bags containing a blend of camomile, catnip, peppermint, skullcap, hops and yarrow. Lincoln developed the formula for this relaxing herbal tea which is now used in a hundred institutions. Clients can drink it at will, but must always take it at bedtime. They also practice autonomy by reading their own computerized printouts of urine and breathalyzer tests, for an objective view of progress.

From sitting peacefully together in a group, addicts learn a form of discipline. As treatment effects accumulate, external discipline promotes internal discipline. Actors and athletes know that *behaving as if* can take you a long way toward *becoming*. By inducing clients' self-discipline, acupuncture treatment relieves the clinic worker of assuming the role of guardian or dictator. Staff-client relationships can thus be person-to-person, rather than superior-to-inferior.

This contrasts sharply with the stratified professional tradition that imposes layers of rank on hospitals and related health-care facilities. It also differs from the hierarchical structure in drug-free therapeutic communities which rank members on a ladder of power that new participants must climb in order to "graduate."

The ease of training chemical-dependency workers in detox acupuncture also affects staffing. Acupuncturists, certified drug-abuse counselors whose academic experience may range from some college to completed higher degrees and people with medical training can all acquire the skill as an additional tool for their work. Nobody's background provides a head start; all must learn this particular technique, which includes a calm, detached, but friendly approach to clients. The democratic climate allows clients to concentrate on receiving treatment, rather than on coping with an institutional hierarchy.

The physical setup is another critical part of the Lincoln Detox protocol. Staff members work where clients can see what's going on, which is not only more efficient but also reduces client anxiety.

An important characteristic of acupuncture is that a patient's response to it can be monitored continually and immediately. Practitioners can make treatment-related decisions on the spot without having to wait for weekly committee meetings or decisions from "upstairs" because in this milieu there is, in effect, no "upstairs." This procedure works well for addicted people, who have very little patience and virtually no tolerance for authoritarian rituals. It could also partly explain why in Lincoln-style clinics one sees little of the rowdiness and edgy, aggressive behavior so common at other drug-free treatment programs and conventional methadone programs.

6

ASPECTS OF NADA

Clinicians founded the National Acupuncture Detoxification Association so that others can replicate the process developed at Lincoln Hospital's Acupuncture Clinic.

As an educational extension of work pioneered at the original Lincoln Detox, NADA defines and maintains a standard for training and certifying Acupuncture Detoxification Specialists.

The NADA treatment plan includes daily ear acupuncture, herbal Sleep Mix tea, participation in Narcotics Anonymous, counseling and computerized daily urine tests. The custom in many conventional detox and treatment centers is to give random, surprise urine tests according to a "one slip and you're out" philosophy. NADA's view is that urine testing is a *positive* feature of a substance-abuse clinic. It's like weighing yourself when you're on a diet, an objective measurement of progress.

NADA membership requires completion of didactic and clinical training at the Acupuncture Detoxification Training Institute (ATI) within Lincoln Hospital's Acupuncture Clinic, or other training sites in the United States and abroad, approved by NADA's board of directors. Membership also requires NADA certification as an "Acupuncture Detoxification Specialist." Applicants must sign an ethics form, and pay annual dues. By 1993 NADA had 1,700 members and seven affiliated organizations in other countries.

ATI training is available to addiction treatment programs which include counseling and medical services and want to add acupuncture to their other modalities. ATI faculty members interview candidates to assess their motivation, temperament and willingness to learn detox acupuncture.

Trainees learn principles of ear acupuncture, needling techniques, sterile precautions and the limitations of what they may do. They learn by first inserting needles in cotton, and later progress to practicing on each other.

The training program's apprenticeship phase involves spending four or five mornings a week at Lincoln or another approved clinic for four weeks, or until both the student and clinical supervisor are confident of the candidate's abilities.

Fully trained acupuncturists who want to work in drug treatment programs take the ATI course, as do experienced chemical-dependency workers who want to expand their professional skills. Those with acupuncture training limited to the NADA protocol are supervised by fully trained acupuncturists. (Florida and some other states permit only fully trained acupuncturists to administer chemical-dependency acupuncture.)

NADA-based sites across the country continue to prove that acupuncture-detox treatment is cheap, simple, effective and attractive to clients. NADA's influence is crucial in U.S. communities where Third World conditions persist— where grown men hang out on street corners, despair breeds violence, drugs abound, neighborhoods disintegrate and too many kids drop out of school.

Drug-dependent people often have related health problems. The linkage of intravenous drug use to AIDS is well-known, as is the sexually-transmitted spread of AIDS to non-users. Diseases aggravated by poverty—asthma, heart

disease, pneumonia, high blood pressure, to list a few—
afflict many addicts. Maternal substance abuse accounts for
the rise in congenital syphilis as well as the growing number of infants in neonatal intensive-care wards. These children often remain hospitalized as boarder-babies, and later
enter congested foster-care systems.

The Anti–Drug Abuse Act of 1988 mandated a fifty-fifty
split between enforcement efforts and prevention/treatment
programs. However, prevention and treatment received only
26 per cent of the nearly $10 billion 1990 budget. Enforce-
ment gets the lion's share of resources.

Many NADA members maintain a private general-acu-
puncture practice and also work in programs operated by
city and county hospitals, in jails and prisons and in clinics
supported by non-profit agencies. Like most U.S. acupuncturists, they insist that quality health care is a right, not a
privilege. These pioneers come from many different backgrounds, but they share the same philosophy: addiction is
an illness. In treating this illness acupuncture is a tool, not
a cure. Treatment must be accessible and flexible, focused
on benefiting the client. NADA is concerned with a process, not with a preconceived agenda.

NADA's first large-scale public conference, held in Santa
Barbara, California, in February 1991 addressed people from
various professions and from institutions in which addiction treatment is a necessary part of work with clients. Acupuncturists attended to learn more about problems of
chemical dependency—addictions to a range of illegal and
legal drugs, including alcohol. Staffers from public, private
and non-profit agencies heard from their NADA-affiliate
counterparts how acupuncture benefits programs.

Learning about each other's concerns proved the theme
of the conference, because addiction treatment relates to
different professional disciplines—acupuncture, corporate
management, law, public health, religion, social work and
Western medicine.

In Santa Barbara, acupuncturists, clinic directors and chemical dependency counselors represented NADA–affiliated programs in all stages of development. NADA's founding member, the Acupuncture Clinic of Lincoln Hospital, was the oldest. Minnesota's Hennepin County Chemical Health Division and Oregon's Portland Addictions Acupuncture Center each had several years' history. Florida's stunningly effective Metro-Dade Drug Court, only a year old at the time of the conference, was already the second-largest program using acupuncture in addiction treatment. Some programs were only several weeks old. Representatives also came from prospective centers here and abroad.

Two preconference retreat days were devoted to purposeful but relaxed information exchange. This is the essence of NADA members' professional interaction: field reports from clinics and programs, discussion of research and funding techniques and ongoing colloquy on how best to integrate acupuncture treatment into public-health-care delivery. Forty attendees from some twenty-two NADA–affiliated programs reported on progress and problems.

Many related their experiences of the adversities of setting up new programs; nobody was smug with success.

❖   An RN and acupuncturist reported that the county-run outpatient clinic where she worked with four other acupuncturists saw ninety chemical-dependent clients every day. The clinic used a two-month acupuncture protocol plus treatment at will. Clients received financial help with transportation. In 1990 the staff started treating pregnant women. Of fourteen pregnant clients, three left the program and eleven had drug-free babies.

❖   A Hungarian psychiatrist said that in her country alcoholism is a very big problem, while drug addiction is minor. With a national population of 10,340,000, there were 500,000 alcoholism patients and only 3,000 beds—so her country needs a therapy that saves beds. (In public-health lingo, *bed* or *slot* means the capacity to treat one person as a residential patient, or inpatient.) This doctor would take NADA training before returning to Budapest.

❖ An acupuncturist-counselor worked in an urban West Coast methadone clinic where some clients were on methadone maintenance, some were detoxifying from heroin on a methadone protocol and some were in-from-the-street heroin users. He said that while the administration permitted acupuncture treatment, it was ambivalent: but the clients were enthusiastic. A parole officer had called to tell him how well a client was doing, explaining that the parolee was more relaxed and was giving more clean urine samples since receiving acupuncture.

❖ A Texas program, state-funded and approved, was getting scant local cooperation. Although the money was available, only five clients had been referred to the acupuncture program from a huge pool of 21,000 probationers with drug-related charges.

❖ An acupuncture-based program fifty miles north of Santa Barbara and open six days a week, saw twenty-five to fifty clients per day. Many continued to come after the treatment period was over, even though they had initially regarded acupuncture as a form of punishment.

❖ The director of a private New York clinic reported that in New York State 40,000 people were on methadone, accounting for three-quarters of the drug treatment "slots." His clinic had a licensed acupuncturist on staff. If a client was addicted to three or more drugs—polyabuse is common—the treatment plan would identify one drug as the primary addictive substance. If the client used alcohol, cocaine and heroin, acupuncture treatment was permitted because there is no methadone equivalent for cocaine treatment.

The New York clinic was open six days a week. To get them through the seventh day clients would have press-pins taped to ear points, to be stimulated as directed. Patients took ten daily treatments and were required to attend three self-help groups.

❖ Two men's prisons in a Midwestern state offered

chemical-dependency acupuncture. A twenty-nine-bed unit of the minimum-security prison was conducting a study in which practitioners used five ear points to treat small groups of inmates. Those inmates who had agreed to try acupuncture were randomly assigned to the experimental group or a control group. The latter did not receive acupuncture. Chemically-dependent people charged with sex offenses and drug offenses were treated in the maximum-security prison, the acupuncturist continued.

"We went into the maximum security prison with the staff not wholly for it", she recalled. "They use a high-confrontation technique in counseling. They want a high anxiety level. One of their concerns was that acupuncture *reduces* anxiety. In the maximum-security prison it's an eight-week program, and it was a real achievement to get permission for an open-ended process.

"When I tell people what I do, they react as if they are very impressed; but really, all I do is go in and give acupuncture. Other people did the really hard work of making it possible."

During a break, three women talked about life at their clinics: "And there was the three-year-old who came in carrying her mother's week-old baby. I had to tell her, 'Sit down! With everybody running around here, somebody could bump into you and the baby could be hurt.' You don't give that responsibility to a three-year-old."

"I hear you," said another woman.

"You know, that child, the only thing she called her mother was 'Bitch.' Like, 'Bitch, can I have a soda?' Because that's what she heard at home. I sat her in my office and asked her name. 'Tisha,' she says. 'That's a pretty name, Tisha. Instead of calling your mother Bitch, why don't you give her a pretty name, too?' 'Okay.' 'Mom's a good name for a mother.' 'Okay.' Took three weeks but now she says 'Mom' like the other kids," said Nancy Smalls, LPN. Smalls is Coordinator of Maternal Substance Abuse Services at Lincoln Hospital, whose department treated 5,000 women in the four years since it opened.

At the time of the conference, Patricia Keenan, OMD, was director of San Francisco's Bayview—Hunters Point Acupuncture Program which saw thirty to fifty clients a day. Keenan talked about treating babies of substance-abusing women. "First I hold the baby, walk around with it, then I hand it back to the mother to see how they interact. Then I treat."

"Kids!" said Carole Myers, Smith's Administrative Assistant and a seventeen-year veteran Lincoln staff member at the time. "There's David: he's three, and somehow that kid learned how to use the telephone while his mom's in the treatment room. He calls up, and I hear this little voice, 'Hi, it's David!' Then he hangs up. After the fourth time in one day, I told him, 'Child, I'm working. Every time you call me I have to stop, so how'm I going to get my work done?' Well, the next day, he goes to another phone—I can see where the call's coming from. I come down the stairs, and there's David running back to Nancy's office, trying to make me think he hadn't been anywhere near that other telephone!"[*]

"Gotta tell you about Candy," said Keenan. "Eighteen months old, he follows me around and 'helps' me give treatment. He pretends his finger is a needle."

"They see treatment from the time they're little," said Smalls. "Maybe we're producing a whole new generation of acupuncturists."

Brian McKenna, a dark-haired lanky man was doing lovely slow *tai chi* near the end of the boardwalk. John Tindall, NADA Coordinator for Great Britain, did a different form on the firm wet sand. (*Tai chi* flickers in the landscape wherever acupuncturists congregate.) These two didn't watch each other, but some comparable moves occurred

---

[*]Carole Meyers died in January 1994.

simultaneously. They stopped at the same time.

McKenna was born in New Jersey and at the time of the conference lived with his wife and two young children in Austin, Texas, where for some years he had a private acupuncture practice. "I went to a lecture about the benefits of acupuncture in HIV-positive people. I thought, this is terrific, but I can't *sell* it, I'd have to give it away."

At a church where an AIDS support group met, McKenna told the group about acupuncture treatment and said that if people were interested, he would contribute four hours per week. Clients would have to find money for needles and supplies. The Austin Immune Health Clinic opened in this church in the spring of 1988 with a budget of about $2,000 and volunteer staff. Six patients came the first week; twelve the following week.

"That first year we figure we delivered $125,000 worth of services on a budget of $6,000," McKenna said. Three years later, at another location, the Immune Health Clinic saw eighty people a week, with a 260-client caseload—half the cases in Austin.

"I have to do administration, which at the beginning I said I wouldn't do, because the clinic has developed beyond the scope of a purely clients-and-clinicians operation. I write protocols [here the word means designs for shaping clinical data] and apply for grants. It's important to tend to the program's health."

Aside from providing a living, McKenna's private practice was a refreshing exercise of his healing art in treating assorted general health problems. At the time of the conference he was still giving four hours a week, his original commitment, to the Austin Immune Health Clinic, which flourished, McKenna says, because of contributions by many people. "I'm not the hero."

NADA attracts talented people for whom the organization is a way of enlarging the scope of work in which they are already engaged. Father Mark Pemberton, a priest of the Russian Orthodox Church in America, and acupuncturist, was NADA coordinator for Texas and New Mexico before his death in 1992.

A few years earlier Pemberton had been working in Austin with McKenna, who invited him along to visit Lincoln. At the time Pemberton was co-chair of the Austin AIDS Interfaith Network, a clergy group. "After three weeks at Lincoln my missionary compassion was aroused by seeing people who really needed something, and were getting it."

London's John Tindall has brought acupuncture to officials as well as to clients. Historically, England has been more open than the United States to complementary medicine, a term embracing acupuncture as well as homeopathy—a therapy favored by members of the royal family. Malpractice insurance for acupuncturists is relatively inexpensive, £160 (about $320) per year. As Tindall says, "If you take training, and get your own insurance, you just go out and do it. A lot of [British] hospitals have acupuncture clinics for pain control. The European Community will probably change health regulations: continentals must be medical doctors to practice acupuncture. But we're an island. We have this attitude that nobody outside should tell us what to do. Besides, too many people want it."

Even with England's greater tolerance for acupuncture, Tindall's achievements typify NADA's energy, tenacity, and ability to navigate around official obstacles.

Tindall's interest in acupuncture was rooted in martial arts training, which he began when he was seven. One teacher, Japanese, also did *shiatsu*, a massage therapy using acupuncture principles.

Qualified as a physiotherapist and having from time to time studied *shiatsu*, reflexology, iridology and Western and Chinese herbalism, Tindall took the two-year licensing course at the British College of Acupuncture, and in 1986, when he was twenty-five, completed the advanced bachelor's degree course.

Tindall was hired as a physiotherapist by St. Thomas's Hospital, one of London's main teaching hospitals, which is linked to satellite hospitals and associated centers. (On Britain's National Health plan, services are free to clients.)

Most of Tindall's career has been with the West Lambeth Health Authority, which encompasses Brixton, a poor South London district similar in quality-of-life to the South Bronx. Brixton has a large black West Indian population and many Asians, including people from Bangladesh, Pakistan, Korea and the Philippines. Brixton had a large drug-dependency clinic treating with methadone, without counseling. When Tindall proposed to add *shiatsu*, iridology, *tai chi* and acupuncture to the program, the authority let him do everything except acupuncture.

Tindall wanted to see what China was doing about addiction in 1987; but people who had been to China told him that nothing noteworthy was going on there. As drugs were illegal, addicts were more apt to go to prison or be executed than receive treatment. Then Tindall saw an article by Michael Smith and wrote to him, explaining that he could get a study grant from Brixton Hospital to learn about the Lincoln Detox program.

Tindall's three-month apprenticeship at Lincoln began in April 1988. He didn't miss a day, and wherever Smith went to speak or give workshops, Tindall went along, paying close attention to his concepts of what makes a clinic work. Tindall traveled to Chicago and conducted NADA training at Pine Ridge Reservation in South Dakota, making a big impact on the Native American detox workers there. At the end of his stint at Lincoln Tindall agreed to represent NADA in the United Kingdom and Europe.

Back in London he proposed to set up treatment in the Brixton program on the Lincoln model, at a cost of £1000 ($1,700) worth of needles. The hospital agreed, reversing its earlier stand against acupuncture, because the drug unit had been losing clients. (Permission to *treat* with acupuncture was all Tindall received. To get needles more cheaply he began a small business of importing them from China.)

"Within three months I was treating in three clinics—

one psychiatric, one inpatient and one community." (The latter refers to a clinic accepting non-referred walk-in clients.) I have lots of NFA's (people with No Fixed Abode). Either they've got no home, or they don't want to tell you where they're from; none of your business, you don't have to know. I was bicycling all over with boxes of needles in my rucksack. Some days I just had to pedal faster."

The psychiatric clinic treats clients with depression, schizophrenia, psychoses, anxiety, panic attacks, anorexia, bulimia and insomnia. One day a man walked in who said he had been hit by a sword, and had been told his infected arm must be amputated. Treatment with Chinese herbs and acupuncture allowed him to retain his arm.

Still employed as a physiotherapist, Tindall began to train hospital nursing staff in the NADA protocol. The nursing administration objected. His immediate supervisor said Tindall was not putting in enough physiotherapy hours and assigned him to another hospital. The move failed to corral Tindall: working at the new location, closer to one of his clinics, cut down his bicycle commute time.

In February 1989, Tindall and Smith went to Sweden's internationally famous and medically prestigious Karolinska Institute. Karolinska invited Tindall to do a NADA training workshop that October. During a subsequent training session elsewhere in Sweden, Tindall conducted classes 12 hours a day to accommodate both beginning and advanced students. (Scandinavia's drug problem is mostly alcohol related.) These sessions prompted formation of Scandinavian NADA, whose leadership Tindall handed over to Sven Wahlstrom, the personnel director of Sweden's National Television. Wahlstrom was another former Lincoln volunteer.

Princess Diana officiated at the 1989 opening of Tindall's Chinese medical service AIDS clinic. When he invited her to experience acupuncture, she asked, "Why, do you think I need it?" "No, but I've always wanted to be able to say, 'By Appointment to Her Majesty,' " Tindall replied. In its first year, this clinic enrolled 149 clients, whose treatment includes acupuncture, Chinese herbs, Chinese diet, and *tai chi* and *qi gong* exercise.

In describing his work Tindall emphasizes the importance of client education and involvement. For example, the clinics he supervises provide herbal teas, and clients have the responsibility of letting staffers know when their supplies of herbal teas are low. Herbs are easy to buy in England, and Tindall's clinics run biweekly herbal seminars so that clients can continue to treat themselves after leaving the program. Detox Tea is the same formula as Lincoln's Sleep Mix. Tindall has formulated his own version of Sleep Tea as well as a kidney tea, a lung tea, a tea for women's cycle problems and a digestive tea.

The West Lambeth Health Authority told Tindall that his acupuncture and related methods saved £80,000 ($156,000), a sum which did not accrue to Tindall's clinics but did to other facilities. Therefore to meet increased demand for services Tindall enlisted the help of "some very altruistic acupuncturists—they wanted to study with me, and in exchange they give services twice a week. In private practice, with the prices they charge, they can do very well seeing only five patients a day. So it's great experience to work in the clinic and treat so many people."

On annual visits to the United States Tindall brings colleagues to NADA conferences and centers. In London he lectures at Guy's Hospital and St. Bartholomew's Hospital—an indication of increased official approval of his work. His job title, Chinese Medicine Specialist in Substance Abuse and AIDS, finally matches his work.

During the Santa Barbara conference's retreat evenings, field reports provided topics for problem-solving in small groups. Here five acupuncturists—three women and two men from programs in different states—shared experiences of bringing acupuncture into conventional drug- and alcohol-treatment programs.

"The day treatment coordinating counselor [at a hospital with a three-week old NADA program] is open to acupuncture, but she's not yet aware of its threat to her counseling approach," one said.

"At our program, counselors never figured bringing in acupuncture might threaten what they actually do," said another.

"The prevailing 'war stories' and rap-session style of counseling is very ineffective. One of our counselors came up with the idea of giving clients a thought to contemplate during treatment, for group discussion later," another reported.

"It's a problem to get them to revolve the whole program around acupuncture as a focus instead of counseling as a focus," a participant pointed out.

"But the diversion program, the one that Miami's known for, uses very little counseling intervention. If they come in and the urines are clean, and they don't seek out their counselor, they can go on home. And it's phenomenally successful," said one of the practitioners.

"Most counselors in nonacupuncture programs spend a lot of time confronting denial. Then, with acupuncture, the substance of discourse changes. This is disconcerting to counselors used to a different style of interaction with clients. Instead of all this confrontational group stuff, people are really working on some problems," someone said.

"[At your place] do they *have* to go to a certain number of group counseling sessions? And then *have* to come to a certain number of acupuncture sessions?" one practitioner asked another.

"No, acupuncture is optional. The day-outpatients are gone by the time we get there. Five-fifteen is the end of their day and they can't wait to get out," was the reply. "We get a better response from evening outpatients because we're the first phase of their evening. They come in at five-fifteen and start with the treatment."

Visiting local acupuncture clinics was part of the conference program. After hearing about intricacies of applying an unconventional healing art in complex circumstances, it was instructive to experience a clinic's apparent simplicity.

Project Recovery was located across town from the conference site. Funded by city, foundation and private money, this acupuncture-based program began seeing clients in 1988, offering treatment for two hours in the morning and afternoon. By the time of the conference, the center had expanded to two locations, employed three acupuncturists, had established a Spanish-speaking Narcotics Anonymous (NA) group, and received cooperation from local criminal-justice personnel. The clinic at 133 East Haley Street was open part-time seven days a week. The second clinic, in a community center, was open for an hour each weekday morning. Unemployed clients were asked to pay what they could; working clients were charged on an income-based sliding scale.

Acupuncture clients were invited to come to the Drop-In Center at East Haley Street to talk about recovery problems, and get assistance and information about issues affecting their lives.

Like many detox and treatment centers, Project Recovery was in a part of town not advertised in tourism brochures. The clinic shared a small wooden single-story building with the Santa Barbara Council on Alcoholism and Drug Abuse. The acupuncturist on duty welcomed four visitors during the conference, including two Hungarian women doctors. She arranged for them to enter the treatment room one-by-one at five-minute intervals and take treatment, so as to observe without disturbing clients

An information sheet set the tone: "You are welcome here and there are no special requirements to enter our program." Enrolled clients picked up two color-coded cards. On one, the client would check off responses to the previous treatment—"worse feeling, no effect, slight relief, great relief"—with regard to thirteen symptoms: "hard to sleep, body aches, headaches, nausea, stomach cramps, sweats, constipation, diarrhea, shakes, cravings, anxiety, drug dreams, depression," and any others not listed. Clients left the treatment-record card on a table for the acupuncturist, who treated in the order of arrival. Each patient cleaned his or her own ears with alcohol-soaked cotton swabs, and sat down in one of the room's eleven chairs. The acupuncturist deftly inserted five needles in each ear.

Three men seated across the room from the visitors addressed each other in Spanish, switching automatically to English when the acupuncturist approached. One wore a baseball hat with an embroidered motto: "Instant Asshole, just add alcohol." On his left was a middle-aged blonde. A younger woman entered accompanied by her thirteen-year-old daughter who sprawled comfortably on the floor reading a book while her mother had treatment. Clients were soft-spoken and composed, at ease with the procedure. The clinic was calm and peaceful, illuminated by fading afternoon light. Forty-five minutes later, following the example of clients who preceded them, the four visitors asked the acupuncturist to remove their needles.

On Friday night, 200 people of many different ethnic and national origins filled the hotel's conference room. It was a professionally diverse congregation, too: acupuncturists, administrators, appointed officials, chemical-dependency workers, doctors of Chinese medicine, MDs and public-agency staff members from across the country.

Familiarity with the recent history of acupuncture in the United States is no preparation for hearing seven men from the fundamentally conservative criminal justice system extol its use. It is astonishing.

Santa Barbara Police Chief Richard Breza was one member of this group. Another was Dennis Shaughnessy, chief administrative officer of Santa Barbara County Probation. The others included Rogelio Flores, Santa Maria's municipal court commissioner, Orville Pung, Minnesota's commissioner of corrections, James Bruton, director of Minnesota's office of adult release (parole), Mark Cunniff, executive director of the National Association of Criminal Justice Planners, and The Honorable Herbert Klein, a circuit judge and the drug czar of Dade County. All had been on the job through changing times and conflicting policies about addict crime management.

Breza, on his return to Santa Barbara from the Portland Addictions Acupuncture Center (Hooper Foundation) said he was called a social worker by colleagues for his interest in getting acupuncture approved.

Shaughnessy, talking about the role of probation and its interface with acupuncture, gave an accurate thumbnail sketch of official policy toward offenders. "The early 1970s was a time when rehabilitation was in. Then about ten years ago intensive supervision came in—'tail 'em, nail 'em and jail 'em.' "

In Santa Barbara County 90 percent of municipal court cases are substance-abuse related. Commissioner Flores found the idea of treating first-offender public inebriates with acupuncture "rather novel" but interesting. "At first I was skeptical—it seemed about as effective as shooting down a B-52 with a pea-shooter." For two years, Santa Maria Municipal Court had been letting first offenders choose between ten days in jail plus a $200 fine, or going to Recovery Point for treatment. Among those choosing the program, the success rate—individuals who have not been rearrested—is over 50 percent. Flores told the group that daily in his court he asked every fourth or fifth defendant's opinion of the bilingual acupuncture program. He has gotten no adverse responses.

Corrections Commissioner Pung deadpanned, "If five years ago someone had told me I'd be in Santa Barbara talking about acupuncture, commitment proceedings would have begun." (Eighty-five percent of Minnesota's inmates have chemical dependency problems.) Pung says of his own experience with NADA-related programs, "After thirty-seven years, to discover a whole new thing is wonderful."

James Bruton was persuasive in discussing the benefits of acupuncture-detoxification. "I've probably said a hundred times, if you have any doubts, go see the clinic at Lincoln, and talk to the people, and ask them why they're there."

Mark Cunniff was blunt about problems in the criminal justice system. Much of his work concerned sentencing and probation in major urban areas. The years 1986 through 1988 saw a 56 percent increase in drug traffickers. Unfortunately, given the large numbers of prisoners with drug problems, there's a sense that treatment people aren't on the same side as criminal justice people.

"The whole concept of rehabilitation took a nosedive in the mid-'70s," said Cunniff. "State treatment people talk to people at the federal level, but at the county level, how do you make contact with the state?"

On the question of proposing new ideas, he said, "The criminal justice system does not talk to itself, let alone to outsiders."

During the George Bush administration, Director William Bennett's Office of National Drug Control Policy was very anti-acupuncture.

Cunniff provided a revealing view of the evolving relationship between criminal justice and treatment. For a workable diversion program—an alternative to incarceration—"you need the cooperation of the prosecutor and of the public defender. Most objections come from the public defender. The thinking is: If the offer comes from the government, it can't be good for my client. "

Los Angeles County Probation has 88,000 people under supervision, 44,000 of whom are drug users. An eighteen-month effort has finally raised money for a treatment program with acupuncture in LA County.

Cunniff continued, "We have invested a lot of money on drug testing in this country, and it does not serve the system." The cost of a drug test for criminal justice use starts at $35 and climbs. It is costly to ensure the chain of custody required when the test is to be used as evidence in court.

He compared high-cost drug testing here with radically simpler methods used, for example, in Singapore which has twenty-five halfway houses for people leaving prison with drug problems, and Malaysia, which has ninety-five such halfway houses.

"We take food, martial arts, cars and money from Asia and it's good quality," said Cunniff. "The only thing we don't take is health care, and look how we're doing with that."

"Crack cocaine really started in Dade County," said Judge Herbert Klein. As a result of 53,000 felony arrests, the county's jail population at the time of the conference was 5,500, with only 4,500 beds. Overcrowded jails lead to a revolving-door system: either more people plea-bargain out of jail sentences, prisoners are released early—regardless of their crimes—or congestion intensifies conditions that produce riots. None of these approaches addresses the problem of the addicted criminal.

In 1989 Klein's superior, Chief Judge Gerald Wetherington, told him they needed a master plan to cope with Dade County's drug problem. Klein explained that drug abuse requires tough, disciplined interdiction as well as treatment; but treatment as yet was unavailable.

Treatment works, Judge Klein told the group, and a person with plenty of money can go to a good program. But large segments of our society have been written off where treatment is concerned.

Given a year off the bench to explore the treatment field and devise Dade County's master plan, Judge Klein traveled all over the United States. At last he visited Lincoln, whose program greatly impressed him. Then he sent Mae Bryant, director of Dade County's Office of Vocational Rehabilitation. She and her associates affirmed his opinion of Lincoln.

As a result, Miami's drug court, which sentences appropriate defendants to treatment using the NADA protocol, was established in record time.

Judge Klein concluded, "You have to have a treatment program that allows clients to steady themselves and have discipline. For many of these people, it's the first time anybody's said, 'we're interested in you.' "

That's not classical law enforcement talk. But for many Americans the criminal justice system is the first point of contact with social services such as addiction treatment, child welfare, health care, psychiatric treatment, vocational training and support in completing high school. So it seems logical and appropriate for a police chief, a judge and other experienced criminal justice professionals to speak like social workers.

This became increasingly apparent in the panels, presentations and workshops at the conference that covered such topics as acupuncture-related research, Chinese medicine in the treatment of AIDS, criminal justice, establishment of a unique residence for HIV-positive people in New York City, fatal child abuse, maternal substance abuse and drug-affected infants, pediatric acupuncture, and the status of NADA programs in the United States and Europe.

All these topics impinge on criminal justice territory. The conference showed that by applying acupuncture to substance-abuse treatment, professionals trained to see addiction as a law-enforcement issue can effectively form an alliance with those trained to see it as a health-care matter.

7

FRONTIERS AND PIONEERS

Acupuncture-based treatment's expansion into new domains is often crippled by American culture's resistance to acupuncture. Thus, a mandate from the top, as in Florida's Dade County program, is a tremendous impetus to success. Dade County's drug arrests and the resultant overcrowding of jails were the dramatic circumstances that spawned Miami's diversion program. As Judge Klein stated, the master plan was formed at a high judicial level and endorsed down the line. Nevertheless, individual counselors and correctional officers balked at change, wanting to protect their own professional turf. Miami acupuncturists had to be diligent, imaginative and generous to win over staff and gain active cooperation. In closed communities like prisons and hospitals, authority figures' passive resistance has a powerfully negative effect.

Mae Bryant, the dynamic director of Dade County's Office of Rehabilitative Services describes this situation.

First of all, correctional officers believe everybody in jail should be in jail and should not be getting treatment in jail, because after all they have committed a crime. Our [existing, nonacupuncture] program in the jail was eighty-five beds. Overnight we went not only to acupuncture, we went to 227 beds at one location.

Not only did we have to deal with counselors who were already in place, we also had to deal with correctional officers. We took the initiative to say, "We want this program to work, so we're going to be the people who take the bigger steps to bring you on with us."

Acupuncturists treated correctional officers at the ungodly hours when they got off their shifts. And allowed them to bring their relatives in who had back pain—those kinds of things. We went beyond the call of duty because that was the only way we could bring the program together.

Acupuncturist Dr. Janet Konefal, associate professor and director of the University of Miami's Master of Public Health program exemplifies "going beyond the call of duty." Dade County hired Konefal to develop the program, which began with in-jail drug treatment and expanded to include an outpatient clinic attached to Drug Court. Konefal's determined efforts on the program's behalf included traveling to treat key personnel with acupuncture before and after her official working day.

As Bryant says, "It's hard, bringing everybody on board. But once you've brought them on board, you never have to say a word about your program, because they sell it for you. The correctional officers would have a *riot* before they allowed us to take the program out of the setting."

Public health revolutions often start as a volunteer effort; but a successful program develops requirements that only reliable funding can ensure. Individual projects apply for support to public agencies, which in turn derive money and power from larger entities. Alcohol, drug and mental health agencies, for example, compete for U.S. Department of Human Services funds.

Numbers make a difference. Officials often dismiss a small clinic's application, claiming that treating a very limited number of clients sheds too little light on how a new method might work on hundreds of clients. On the other hand, large numbers of needy people can swamp an experimental new effort which lacks both a sturdy financial base and political interest in its survival.

When a therapy still regarded as radically unusual joins an existing treatment program, intramural strains often appear. Hierarchically minded workers resist adopting a more flexible and open work-style with each other and with clients.

A program that is and always has been acupuncture-based is more likely to succeed, but harder to fund.

Initial enthusiasm by program directors or local authorities does not always produce a flourishing clinic or program. Many factors affect success or failure, including uncontrollable variables like good luck and timing. A project carefully nursed into existence in an institution which merely tolerates it might then fade away—and years later, when circumstances have changed the same institution might welcome a similar project.

During the winter of 1984–1985 there was talk of establishing an acupuncture clinic in Gouverneur, on the northeastern edge of New York's Chinatown. Gouverneur is the primary ambulatory health care center for an ethnically mixed population; at that time the mix included Jews, Italians, and Chinese. The clinic was not yet operational, but visitors were allowed.

A few red and gold Chinese New Year signs and some framed classical Chinese art posters decorated the reception area. The medical director, psychiatrist Dr. Wen Yeung, studied acupuncture in 1968 while attending the University of Hawaii. His mother, "an old-fashioned Chinese lady," did not approve of his taking evening acupuncture classes. One day she suffered some pain and weakness. He applied heat with a hair dryer to a leg point. His mother's problem disappeared, and with it her objections to his acupuncture studies.

Yeung, who maintained a private practice Saturdays and some evenings, worked half-time at a Chinatown community health center and half-time at Gouverneur. He explained why acupuncture was being offered at the Asian Mental Health Clinic, a unit of Gouverneur's psychiatric service. "For Chinese with psychiatric problems there seems to be a higher component of somatic problems than in whites." Clientele would be primarily Chinese and other Asians. The hospital did not propose to expand acupuncture to other populations.

By the spring of 1992 this had changed, and Gouverneur had developed an acupuncture program with slots for six staff members. Coordinating manager Pamela King considers this group a team rather than a hierarchy. Other staff members are Walter Bosque, acupuncturist and addiction counselor, bilingual in Spanish and English; social worker Lorraine Koenig, and administrative assistant/receptionist Amy Kan, who is fluent in several varieties of Chinese as well as in English. A licensed acupuncturist and a psychiatrist were still being recruited. King and Koenig took chemical-dependency acupuncture training at Lincoln Detox in the spring of 1991. Bosque, trained in acupuncture and with a degree from the Acupuncture Association of Quebec, worked at Lincoln Detox from the time the clinic was methadone-based through the early acupuncture period, until 1979.

Gouverneur Hospital never had a formal substance abuse program. It now has one, albeit minimal, offering acupuncture detox but no related social services. For AA and NA groups, clients must go elsewhere.

The acupuncture program is on the fourth floor. A U-shaped space open to the corridor serves as its reception area and leads to two offices and two treatment rooms. The clinic is bright and cheerful, with butter-yellow walls and lavender trim. Each treatment room accommodates several clients at once. They occupy padded tables or straight chairs. Three different in-hospital clinics refer clients to the acupuncture program: the Dr. Daniel Leicht assessment clinic for HIV–positive people, the psychiatric clinic, and the obstetrics and gynecology clinic. All clients receive a brief description of acupuncture with details of its effects on HIV/ AIDS, substance abuse and stress reduction. (Stress and anxiety are common factors in the first two conditions.)

Treatments began in May 1991, although there was a one-week interruption when everybody was laid off during the city's budget crisis. The program really got off the ground in late July. Nine months later the program was seeing twenty-five people a day; the hospital administration's goal is forty when a larger space becomes available. Random urine tests are given, using a temperature-strip. (Variations from body temperature reveal adulteration.) These tests indicate client progress or relapse, but are not valid for court matters. After years of experience King says, "Clients would think you were a fool if you didn't test urines."

Chemically dependent clients involved with parole, probation or child welfare are mandated to enroll in some substance-abuse treatment program but they are not directed to any specific one. Each decides which program he or she will attend. Gouverneur Acupuncture Clinic clients are mostly Hispanic, then non-Hispanic white, then black, and a few Asians.

Individual counseling takes place when a client requests it. Koenig says that staffers can suggest counseling to a client but most often counseling is a matter of crisis intervention, not a long-term plan. Fees are on an income-based sliding scale. Medicaid pays for indigent clients.

Two women who have just finished treatment are typical Gouverneur clients. One says she is been off methadone for twenty-one days after fifteen months on methadone maintenance. "If I don't leave now, I'd beat your eardrums talking about it," the other says with a smile. A few minutes later, pushing her two-year-old daughter in a stroller, another arrives for treatment. She is young and pretty and

HIV-positive, and says that acupuncture really helps the stress.

Walter Bosque, in his forties, comes from the South Bronx. One of the founders of the Young Lords was a friend of his. Bosque was going to nursing school when Lincoln Detox started, and his friend told him to come and look, "and I started volunteering."

Bosque's interest in acupuncture began with studying *tai chi*. This martial art is a common introduction to acupuncture for Occidentals because *tai chi* instructors—Asian or non-Asian—often allude to other aspects of Asian culture. Bosque was one of the five Lincoln Detox workers awarded the Doctor of Acupuncture degree in 1979.

After the Koch bust of 1979, Bosque was assigned to another city hospital. For several years he taught at the Tri-State Institute of Traditional Chinese Acupuncture, where he was Assistant Director. His work at Gouverneur began in 1990, when the acupuncture program was still in development. With a classically wry New York City view of reality, Bosque says, "It only took about six years to get this thing going."

Both rural and urban civic environments may, for murky political reasons, prove hostile to an innovative program, though this hostility is detrimental to individual human needs. Carol Taub is a Los Angeles acupuncturist and NADA boardmember who for years has divided her time between public health and private practice. Now she works in a county jail program and also at the Asian American Drug Abuse Program (ASDAP) treating pregnant women and mothers in a multicultural neighborhood.

Starting in November 1986, Taub directed Turnaround Alternative Treatment Program, a walk-in addiction treatment center for homeless people. Operating on Los Angeles' Skid Row, Turnaround was a volunteer-run demonstration project. (A demonstration project is intended to show that the work is effective and valuable enough to be funded as an operating program.) Before going to their regular jobs, volunteer acupuncturists, counselors and administrators put in their stint at Turnaround, which was open in the mornings for about eighteen hours a week. In its fourteen months of existence more than 1,600 homeless men and women used the program. This seems a sturdy enough demand for services to ensure the program's viability. Yet in January 1988, Turnaround was obliged to close because the city-donated building had been promised to another program, a center for mentally ill homeless people. This occurred although health services in the huge Los Angeles County were in great decline.

Two weeks before Turnaround shut its doors, three television channels covered the story. Clients told what Turnaround had done to help them shake off addiction. Staff members spoke movingly about the clinic's value. A few city officials delivered verbal parachutes of praise. But this media wake did not resuscitate the project.

Taub says Turnaround was one of the only walk-in centers that accepted everyone who asked for help. Referring to its demise, she addresses a classic dilemma: "Why does one good program have to die because there is another needy one?"

Public-health centers function differently in different states and countries. Minnesota's longstanding concern for social justice perhaps stems from the traditionally egalitarian culture of the state's many citizens of Scandinavian descent. Minnesota was the first state to push for insurance coverage of addiction patients—a move that meant the state's residential chemical-dependency treatment centers were a substantial business.

Robert Olander, academically trained in social psychology, is director of Hennepin County's Chemical Health Division. In 1981, Blue Carstenson, an acupuncture advocate, and Patricia Culliton, an acupuncturist, called and introduced him to the concept of treating narcotics and methadone addicts with acupuncture. Olander then read publications by Smith and the Lincoln team along with other relevant materials.

"I'd been around the clinical scene—methadone, talk therapy—for about twenty years. There were many clients not doing well. I said, 'come on over, let's see what we can do with it.' We did an in-service demonstration on patients."

The chemical health division's medical director, Milton Bullock, thought the technique might work with other populations too. The county was running a major detox center for chronic alcoholics. What intrigued Bullock were results on the two intractable factors, withdrawal and long-term psychological craving.

Olander explains that Minnesota's well-known established programs were all built around AA's 12-Step model—elaborated from AA but nevertheless holding to AA tenets, one of which is to avoid therapies that substitute one drug for another. There were three major hindrances to acupuncture's success here. First, the state had a very public, powerful model. Next, doctors were uninterested in observing acupuncture demonstrations. And third, even the most creative people felt that clinical work was not as strong a proof of therapy's validity as standard research methods. Research was needed.

The research came in a pilot study of alcoholic recidivism by Milton Bullock, Andrew J. Umen, MS, Patricia D. Culliton, MA, and Olander. That study offers a clear picture of the contemporary situation.

"Acupuncture is presently being used by a number of clinics in this country to treat alcohol and drug-addicted individuals, but despite encouraging results, it has not achieved widespread acceptance as a useful modality in the treatment of addictive disorders. Efforts to encourage its use as an effective, yet inexpensive, form of treatment have been hampered by skepticism engendered by the exotic nature of the procedure, the lack of understanding of its mechanism of action, and by the absence of controlled studies of treatment of alcohol and drug addiction."

As a medical doctor, however, Bullock could muster

some political support. With this pilot study, Olander recalls, "We began to be a research source, giving Western medical validity to chemical-dependency acupuncture. We used the research model to affirm Mike Smith's clinical model. By the mid-1980s Lincoln was seeing 100, 200, or 300 clients a day. There were hundreds of successful anecdotal cases, people who never had responded to traditional treatment. In 1983–1984 we hoped to make the leap from a pilot project to a broader population and type of craving. We did a more defined study."

This eighty-patient study, titled "Controlled Trial of Acupuncture for Severe Recidivist Alcoholism," was carried out from December 1986 to October 1987. Although not published until 1989—in the prestigious British medical journal *Lancet*—data from the study circulated among treatment professionals.

That broke the local logjam. Even the more skeptical institutional people started to say that maybe something was happening. At the same time, crack, the cheap, swiftly addictive, smokable form of cocaine, emerged as a substance as intractable as alcohol.

"Forces seemed to be gathering," Olander recalls. Treatment centers all over the country were finding that people on crack were not responding to any conventional therapy, while more and more people were apparently doing well with the NADA protocol. "Crack convinced many reluctant administrators to try the NADA treatment method."

Begun with a phone call to a county health program director from two individuals, Hennepin County's acupuncture involvement grew tremendously in ten years, advancing one step at a time with close ties to clinical research. Hennepin County Community Services Department, Chemical Health Division Acupuncture Program is a freestanding acupuncture service with clients referred from seven community programs. Pat Culliton, director of acupuncture, has a corrections research project: acupuncture both in prison and with community probation.

"One thing we're looking at is, how many treatments, for how long: week, day, hour? Dose response: five treatments on a daily basis, or twice a week, or three times?" says Olander. (Dose response is a topic of investigation in pharmacological research.)

Patricia Culliton, Dipl.Ac., is one of NADA's founding board members. She had for some years been chief acupuncture researcher and member of Hennepin County Medical Center's medicine department when she spoke to a professional audience about acupuncture research.

"I attempted to do research in 1981, but it took us two years before we could treat our first person, and it was not until 1987 that we actually saw our data in print." (In 1995, Culliton received a major research grant from the NIH's Office of Alternative Medicine.)

The capacity to produce research can improve a clinic's financial health. In order to generate research results, a program can lend itself to observation by outsiders, or develop its own research project. Clinical researchers must often tailor their designs to the understanding of funding-agency officials, who naturally think in terms of Western medical research. As one experienced administrator said about designing acupuncture research, "You have to speak the language of the occupying army."

Another pressure on research design is the reluctance of policymakers in one part of the country to accept acupuncture data accumulated in other states. The director of a treatment center in a state where acupuncture is relatively new secured substantial funding for his program by writing a grant proposal involving research which duplicates investigations already amply documented in other states. His state will not accept out-of-state studies as a basis for action. By securing the research grant he nevertheless makes it possible to treat clients in the program.

Innovative public health work needs constant affirmation in order to continue. It is difficult for smaller centers to do the research that will support their program's validity. Documenting clients and their treatment is normal routine.

But determining what information to extract from clinical records—or designing treatment which illuminates a particular aspect of acupuncture in substance abuse—are other tasks. Writing proposals to secure funding with which to hire those who can do such work is yet another job. Larger clinics are more able to allocate staff time to the kind of paperwork which ensures continued existence.

The hard fact is that acupuncture research allows policymakers to see with other people's eyes. And compilation of data makes a paper shield for their decisions.

Even so, the most effective encounters between government officials or bureaucrats and acupuncturists wishing to demonstrate the therapy occur when policymakers agree to receive a sample treatment. Arriving at a program site, they bustle in with briefcases, prepared for adversarial negotiations. Accepting a few judiciously placed needles, they relax and tend to remove their jackets, sit on the floor and not only talk to one another, but also listen.

If only all officials could learn what happens in group settings by taking treatment along with chemically dependent clients . . . but that's about as realistic as expecting New York City's mayor to ride the subway regularly.

8

THIRD WORLD NATIONS, USA

Although Lincoln's ear-acupuncture treatment for drug dependency began with heroin addicts, from the earliest days Lincoln's acupuncture program detoxified alcoholic clients as well, and in twelve years accumulated a solid record of inducing early sobriety. The effect on alcohol addiction is now being seen on Indian reservations where the treatment has been introduced.

Like inner-city ghettoes, many Indian reservations are places of despair and thwarted human potential, where lethal poverty levels destroy hope. Such poverty produces high rates of accidental death and deaths from heart disease as well as chronic obstructive pulmonary diseases like emphysema, respiratory diseases like pneumonia and influenza, adult diabetes, chronic liver disease and alcohol-induced cirrhosis.

Along with dismal economic prospects, alcoholism is the bane of Native American enclaves, the primary drug of dependency even when other drugs are used. Indian Health Service statistics for 1990–1992 showed Native Americans dying from alcohol-related causes at 5.5 times the rate of the United States' population as a whole.

The ravages of alcohol abuse have extensive consequences: preventable but irreversible Fetal Alcohol Syndrome (FAS) causes some unborn children to be developmentally damaged by alcohol toxicity in the mother's bloodstream. Physical evidence of these damages include abnormal head size, low-set ears, broad nosebridge, underdeveloped cheekbones and smooth, thin upper lip. Ear, eye, kidney and respiratory problems often afflict these children as they grow. Some are retarded. Some develop behavioral problems.

Studies have shown that from 5 to 25 percent of reservation-born children are born with FAS. These children endure a double blow: in addition to their own abnormalities, they have mothers too sick from drinking to nurture them adequately. These children are difficult to place in either foster or adoptive homes. Children with FAS have been identified in Europe and in the general American population—one estimate puts worldwide incidence under one percent. FAS is not race-specific, but its prevalence in the impoverished Native American population of 1.9 million is just one more indignity.

Adult alcoholism also takes an emotional toll on growing children. The bill comes due in adolescence, an uneasy state even under the best of conditions. A study of youth health commissioned by the Indian Health Service, carried out by the University of Minnesota and published in 1992 in the *Journal of the American Medical Association* revealed profoundly sad youngsters whose circumstances drain away any optimism. The rate of drinking problems in young Native American teenagers increases with time. The study also notes that the suicide rate among American Indian and Alaska Native youth (26.3 per 100,000) is double that of other groups of the same age in the United States.

Alcoholism, dying infants, FAS-damaged children and profoundly despondent youths, all in one racial group, sounds like a recipe for genocide. Politics, economics, and questions of tribal autonomy have always affected attempts to treat Native American alcoholism. Conventional treatment involving inpatient detoxification and prescription sedatives like chloral hydrate was never very realistic for Native American clients on rural reservations which, among other hazards, lack detoxification facilities.

Bringing acupuncture to Native Americans is not as great a stretch as it might seem at first glance. Native American observers have remarked on the similarity between acupuncture concepts and their traditional medicine's philosophy of energy flow.

In May–June 1986, at the invitation of tribal health service officials, NADA sent teams to conduct workshops for detox workers in Montana and South Dakota reservation alcoholism programs. The five-person teams were to demonstrate the usefulness of acupuncture detox for Native American clinics and clients. They would teach Native American alcoholism staff the techniques, uses and limitations of NADA's ear acupuncture treatment and they would help implement an acupuncture component in the local alcoholism program.

In the Lincoln Detox tradition, observers were permitted. At Crow Agency visitors included acupuncturists and others from British Columbia, California, New York and Texas.

Crow Agency is a small western crossroads town on the Crow Indian Reservation. It lies just off the highway, 50 miles east of Billings, Montana, where Interstate 90 bends southward to parallel the Little Bighorn River. Custer's Last Stand Cafe, a restaurant and tourist shop, accommodates visitors to Custer Battlefield National Monument⁺ and museum. License plates bear the motto, "Big Sky Country," and as you head out of Billings into emptiness, you see few vehicles and almost no houses as darkness falls. At the Last Stand Cafe, just before the 9 P.M. closing time, if you ask the

---

⁺Officially renamed Little Bighorn National Battlefield in 1992 to commemorate the Battle of Little Bighorn.

waitress at the counter for a much-anticipated beer, mocking laughter sounds from the dim, half-empty area where local people occupy a few booths and tables. Crow Indian Reservation is officially dry—doesn't everybody know that? (Liquor is banned on three-fourths of the United States' 293 reservations. The fact that bootleggers thrive in a dry locality with a high alcoholism rate is not immediately obvious.)

It is election time for the four-member tribal council— chair, vice-chair, secretary and vice-secretary—which governs the reservation and meets three times a year. (Modern tribal government dates from the 1920s.) Women can vote from the age of eighteen; men, from twenty-one. Polls are open from 1 A.M. to 8 P.M. on Saturday. More than thirty candidates compete for these full-time, two-year salaried positions. Signs all over Crow Agency announce election-related "feasts and gatherings."

The weekly *Hardin Herald,* published at the Big Horn County seat, is packed with political advertisements. One office-seeker proposes that the tribe's employees should be hired on merit and work a forty-hour week. Several suggest a switch to the secret ballot. One promises to demand that the Bureau of Indian Affairs (BIA) help to promote tribal goals rather than dictate them. Another outspoken candidate writes that every member of the tribe should participate in tribal government without fear that a vote on the wrong side might endanger employment—either the voter's or a relative's—with the tribe.

Political statements are laced with accusations of nepotism and of fiscal shenanigans, not unusual in insular, economically depressed communities. If you are a police officer, can you handle arresting your uncle for theft? If you work for a child welfare agency, how do you deal with clients accused of alcohol-related child abuse who happen to be in your extended family?

Tribal members campaigning for office publicly deplore the high alcoholism rate and the influx of drugs to the reservation.

At NADA's Crow Agency training sessions, Native American clinicians from regional alcoholism programs planned to learn acupuncture techniques designed specifically to alleviate physical and emotional reactions to withdrawal, and to support recovery maintenance.

Family Services director, Henry Pretty On Top, a slim, fortyish man wearing aviator glasses and well-shined cowboy boots, showed visitors to the Baptist church where they met Archie Bear Ground, director of the Alcoholism Treatment Program at Crow Agency. Inside, the Crow woman in charge, Sonja Stewart, welcomed the strangers despite her disappointment that they were not the NADA team.

The room was about thirty by sixty feet; benches used for church services lined the walls to clear space for training sessions. A couple of trestle tables stood near the door. One held a coffee urn, orange-soda keg and pastries. The other held flyers, photocopied news articles and several clipboards, typical civic meeting appurtenances. A dozen other Native Americans stood around the room speaking in low voices.

Their questions revealed much curiosity and some anxiety about this unusual therapy. An older man remarked. "This acupuncture sounds a little like our traditional healing. The part about energy, and helping the body heal itself."

"My uncle," a woman said. "I don't know why he isn't dead. He's got a mountain of Lysol spray cans all around his house. Punches a hole in the can and lets the Lysol run out and drinks it."

"How old is he?" someone asked.

"About sixty-five."

Estelle Fielder of the Cheyenne River Sioux was visiting Crow Agency. She had recently resigned as director of the Cheyenne River Alcoholism Program in South Dakota. She said it was hard to get funding. People in charge were themselves abusing substances, and the programs threatened them. The church's literature table had photocopies of the Fielder's *Lakota Times* article on alcoholism in which Fiedler wrote, "Alcoholism has been and always will be the number one impediment to the health, economic, social and educational welfare of our people."

Snow sludged down the church windows in large, wet, late-season flakes. Early May was bleak and dank that day in Crow Agency. Weather was delaying the NADA team.

"As long as we get our points for study, I don't mind if they're late," Sonja Stewart commented.

"Your acupuncture points?" asked a visitor.

"Points for study. We need a certain number of points for the state."

"Oh, professional education points." the visitor said. "I thought you meant *acupuncture* points." Stewart laughed.

Orrie Plain Bull said, "Whenever there's an event, a meeting, we always ask what they're providing for refreshment before we decide to go. It may be a cultural thing." His tone was low-key, humorous.

Someone started running a film about teenagers and the dangers of alcohol. It emphasized the risks of drinking and driving—which is a major problem in rural areas without public transportation, where locating liquor can involve long-distance trips.

A man spoke of his difficulty in getting money from the Indian Health Service for substance-abuse work. He thought prevention and treatment should have its own department under the Bureau of Indian Affairs, rather than be subject to IHS.

The snow-spangled NADA team came through the door at four o'clock: training coordinator David Eisen from Somerville, Massachusetts; Tony Huerta and Michael Smith from Lincoln; Pamela Mills from Chicago; and NADA consultant Naomi Lev who had driven from Missoula, Montana, 350 miles away. They shed their coats and set to work, laying out sleep-mix teabags, needles in sterilized packs, alcohol swabs, a plastic mannequin and an oversize model of an ear.

Class began. With the easy manner of someone telling a friend how to tie fishing-flies, Smith reassured the group. "Don't worry about being skeptical," he said. "I was too, at first." He told the participants that they would learn to identify points on the external ear—Shen Men, Sympathetic, Kidney, Liver and Lung—and how to insert needles. During the next hour and a half only a few people held back from the acupuncture experience. Most, including Bear Ground, Stewart and Plain Bull, allowed the teachers to insert needles in their ears.

The team didn't limit its demonstration to the detox technique. Some of the students became patients and were treated on the spot with general medical acupuncture. One man lacked feeling in his fingers, residue of an old driving accident in which his arm smashed through the windshield and was badly cut. A woman and another man asked for treatment of musculoskeletal problems.

Early the next morning still more acupuncturists and tribal health workers gathered in the Baptist church. The new arrivals sat on benches along one side of the room. Yesterday's fellow students greeted each other by name and praised the heating system's improved performance.

Plain Bull asked in a serious manner, "Looking at this [ear] chart, I see back and wrist and things—but what is there for the man whose wife's just left him and taken the kids?"

Students learned that a point named for an organ also deals with emotions connected with that organ: for instance Shen Men is the gate to the spirit, the spirit being what makes you grow; Kidney affects fear, and Liver affects anger and frustration. The workshop alternated needle-technique practice with discussion, acupuncture theory and clinical anecdotes.

Teachers reminded students that they already had experience working with detox patients—acupuncture would be an additional professional tool.

Naomi Lev, RN and acupuncturist, is a transplanted Israeli who had been working with Flathead Indians. The established Flathead alcoholism program was inpatient detoxification. It cost $4,000 to $7,000 per person, and the success rate was 10 percent.

Lev described the community-based outpatient program she designed, which was funded for an initial six months. It involved setting up a clinic and alcoholism center in the Flathead Reservation town of Arlee, about forty miles northwest of Missoula. Tribal health workers would bus clients to Arlee where Lev would treat three times a week. She said that some people with severe DT's had to go to the hospital, but she was able to treat some pretty severe cases of DT's in her office.

Herman White Grass, one of three Blackfoot Indians visiting from Browning, Montana, was dubious about outpatient treatment. To reassure clinical workers about its effectiveness, researchers told students about the three-month study Pat Culliton conducted in Minnesota on fifty-four chronic alcoholics, each of whom had a record of many admissions to the county detox center. The men were assigned to control and experimental groups, given bed and board in a pleasant facility and free bus tokens with which to go downtown. One group received acupuncture at real points, the others at points not specific for chemical dependency. No counseling was given, only acupuncture. As the study progressed, some of the sham-point men would pick fights with the real-point people for not joining them at a bar for a couple of drinks.

Someone asked, "Would you take a patient off chloral hydrate, Librium, or Valium when you're doing acupuncture?"

"Add the acupuncture," is the answer. "Patients will begin not to want the drug."

"How do you get clients to accept acupuncture treatment?"

"Show them peace and quiet in the clinic. They want that." Bear Ground remarked that the first treatment felt so good, he was going to have one every day; maybe it would help his arthritis.

Among themselves, local people generally speak the Crow language. Many Crow people speak English with an accent that sounds Eastern European. The forty-something Herman White Grass says that Crow children here grow up bilingual. In his generation, Browning's Blackfoot children didn't learn their tribal language, but his grandmother taught him some. He can understand Blackfoot but could not speak it as fluently as he would have liked. Now they're talking about getting it into the schools.

The NADA session had become a gathering—people would hear something unusual was going on; they came in and watched for a while, then continued on their way.

Practice began after lunch. Students worked in pairs, with an acupuncturist directing each pair, and tried to locate ear points by lightly touching spots on the outer ear. Sometimes they reported a tiny pulse, like an earthworm's heartbeat.

You hold the needle between thumb and forefinger, set its point against the spot, then push-twist in one smooth move. (Hesitation inflicts pain.) The depth of insertion is about one-eighth of an inch. Houston acupuncturist Phillip Puddy showed how, demonstrating on a man's ear. "Now, you try it," he directed. The needle went in and the man didn't flinch.

At the other end of the table, David Eisen supervised. Sherry LaForge, who the previous day shook her head at the idea of being needled, now had needles in her ears.

In came Henry Pretty On Top. Eisen briefed him. Pretty On Top studied the ear chart, then removed his glasses and, under Eisen's scrutiny, inserted two needles in a woman's right ear.

On Saturday, training moved to the Detox Clinic, formerly a private house. In what must have once been the living room, the team explained that acupuncture induces early sobriety. Sobriety is not enough, but it *is* a beginning.

Acupuncture produces a clearer, calmer person who, in time of trouble, can remember what the therapist said.

When acupuncture was first used at Lincoln, needling was done at different points for different addictions. Then they found that heroin points worked for alcohol, and alcohol points worked for cocaine, though alcohol and cocaine affect the system very differently. They concluded that this is a treatment for *poisoning* rather than for specific drugs. Drugs affect the Jing (seed) energy. Having tried many formulas, they were teaching the most effective one at this workshop. It was and is the formula currently used at Lincoln.

Someone asked if acupuncture was required at Lincoln, and if not, how did staffers persuade clients to try it? At Lincoln, a team member explained, anyone who comes to the clinic is admitted and newcomers are asked if they want acupuncture or counseling. Usually they choose counseling, which is done in the acupuncture room. Clinical workers nodded approval of this common-sense approach to inducing clients to try new treatment.

Practice resumed. White Grass placed a needle in his partner's right ear. She praised his dexterity. This distracted him and he hesitated before pushing in the next one.

"That wasn't as good as the first," he said. The third was fine, and his partner said so.

The supervising acupuncturist remarked, "It's useful to have a responsive patient when you're learning. In detox they don't sit so still."

White Grass slid the next two smoothly into his partner's left ear. Removing needles reveals whether or not they were properly inserted. All these were. White Grass was a diligent student.

A detailed written plan of the treatment process reinforced the training sessions and would guide detox workers once they were on their own. Eisen stayed on for a week and gave 155 treatments, which not only attracted and served clients, but also put the program on a solid footing. After his departure, he called weekly. Naomi Lev was assigned to visit the program regularly to help maintain clinical standards. NADA was a continually available resource while the program gained experience with the new technique.

The Crow Agency NADA sessions had immediate positive results. The number of clients attending the Crow Detoxification Program increased substantially, so that two months after training the program was giving forty acupuncture treatments a week. This was a 500 percent increase over the clinic's number of daily treatments before it incorporated acupuncture.

A June 29, 1986, article in *Montana Territory, The Missoulian*'s Sunday supplement, covered the Crow Agency story. Reporter John Stromnes wrote about Montanan addicts for whom acupuncture treatment proved effective. Acupuncture has been an independently licensed profession in Montana since 1974, but in 1986 its use in detoxification was still news.

Stromnes wrote:

> [M]embers of [NADA] recently helped Crow Indians begin an acupuncture outreach program for alcoholics on the Crow reservation near Hardin.

> "Perhaps 75 percent of the adults on the reservation are alcoholics," said Archie Bear Ground, director of the Crow Tribal Detoxification Program.

> Patients report they feel a sense of profound relaxation, a calming of their nerves, and they lose the desire for a drink for the time being.

> "The needle treatment, plus a special herb tea mix and follow-up counseling, may help many of the Crow control their alcoholism," Bear Ground said. He said the program will continue using its own natural-healing methods—sweat-lodge visits and prayer. [Sweat-lodge is a traditional technique for physical cleansing and meditation.]

> The acupuncture program started in mid-May. In one six-day period last week 34 people took acupuncture treatment instead of the regular detox treatment that involves the use of prescription tranquilizers.

"Right now, it's too early to make an evaluation of the success rate of our [acupuncture] treatment," [Bear Ground] said. He said he will have a better idea by the end of the summer.

But the program has already had an unexpected benefit. Since 1979, Bear Ground has had a chronic hearing problem—a loud ringing in one ear. As part of his training in May, he took five alcohol detox acupuncture treatments.

"I took those five treatments and that ringing sound went away," he said.

Despite this meticulously designed and well-supported beginning, the Crow Agency acupuncture program eventually fell victim to local politics. The 1986 election resulted in changes which in time affected tribal health-care delivery. For reasons unrelated to considerations of its effectiveness, the Crow Agency acupuncture program closed. On another reservation, however, acupuncture programs endure.

South Dakota's Pine Ridge Reservation is the site of Wounded Knee, where in 1890 U.S. soldiers massacred Chief Big Foot and 300 other Sioux captives—men, women and children. It is also where, in 1975, tension of more recent origin between the Federal Government and the American Indian Movement erupted in a firefight in which two FBI agents were killed.

Oglala Sioux inhabit the reservation's nearly two million acres, two-thirds of which lie within Shannon County, which the 1989 census defines as the poorest county in the United States. Statistics give a rock-hard picture of life at Pine Ridge: in 1989 a scant three in ten adults were employed. In 1991, when 14.2 percent of the U.S. population lived in poverty—defined as income under $12,000 for a family of four—Shannon County's poverty rate stood at 63.1 percent. Consequently some adults look for work away from home, leaving children with grandparents or other relatives. Welfare is integral to existence on Pine Ridge Reservation today. As one tribal leader told *New York Times* reporter Peter T. Kilborn (September 20, 1992), " 'We're a fifth- going-on-sixth-generation welfare state.' "

A month after the Crow Agency sessions, a NADA team comprised of Minnesota's Patricia Culliton, and clinicians from Lincoln Hospital—Sonia Lopez, Khunat Ra, training coordinator Priscilla Santiago and Michael Smith—conducted training sessions at Pine Ridge's Project Recovery, an addictions treatment center established in 1972. In addition to alcohol, clients here also abuse cocaine, marijuana and inhalants such as gas and lighter fluid. Polyabuse is common. Project Recovery clients receive free services. The treatment center does not handle medication; when necessary, clients are sent to the hospital for medically supervised detox.

NADA sessions met enthusiastic response, the Pine Ridge *Lakota Times* reported. One hundred and fifty people came to try acupuncture at Project Recovery . "[T]hose who were treated by the New York team weren't all alcoholics. Young and old came for treatment of back problems, sinus and hay fever, arthritis, diabetes, weight loss or because they wanted to quit smoking," the newspaper reporter noted.

This NADA team followed the same procedures as did the Crow Agency team: demonstration, instruction, establishment of the acupuncture component's treatment program, follow-up and supervision. But human and local variables are unpredictable. Seven years later, acupuncture was well-rooted in Pine Ridge.

In 1990, Project Recovery acupuncturist and counselor Sandy Cuny said the center was seeing twenty-five clients a month, aged eleven to sixty. About ten of these came for acupuncture. Half the clients were walk-ins. The rest were referred by the Oglala Sioux Tribal (OST) Court and, in the case of younger clients, by schools. (While some reservation schools, both K-8 and high school, are tribally sponsored, others are BIA-sponsored. Still others are public or parochial.) With parental consent, children received acupuncture. Cuny said the girls and women liked acupuncture, but boys and men were skeptical. Pregnant substance abusers were not receiving acupuncture; meditation, diet and herbal teas were used instead.

With a client who hadn't drunk for a couple of weeks and was struggling against taking a drink, or someone coming in drunk asking for help, Cuny would describe acupuncture and usually the client would allow her to give treatment. She said, "Eight out of ten people who have acupuncture return for more treatment. When a new client appears, I stress that they should come back for three days. I tell them, 'it took a while to get into this state of dis-ease; you can't expect one forty-minute treatment to do the job.' "

Three members of 1990's fulltime staff of eight were NADA-certified: Director Jeaneen Grey Eagle, Cuny and Ila Red Owl. Wayne Weston, a former staffer, was also NADA-certified. Every year NADA sent someone out to recertify them—in 1989 the trainer was the Englishman, John Tindall, who Cuny said inspired those who worked with him.

Project Recovery lacked funding for urine tests, so when such tests were court-ordered, staffers would supervise and send specimens to the lab, and would be reimbursed for six dollars per test.

As at other acupuncture-based centers, clients who dropped out and returned were accepted as long as they felt the need. Project Recovery maintained NADA's group treatment principle, in which five or six clients sat in one room on donated chairs. This branch of acupuncture flowers in poverty.

Project Recovery serves the entire Pine Ridge Reservation. The long distances make daily treatment impractical for some clients. So practitioners inserted not regular two-inch needles but tape-covered press-needles which do not protrude and can be left in place for days at a time. These clients were told to massage the points three times a day for three minutes. Cuny reported that no clients developed infection. On sobriety campouts, people requesting press-needles were asked to make a donation—and most did.

On the topic of treatment success, Cuny said, "When the person can work for spiritual progress, and maintain sobriety and I see that spark in the eye, of effort—it's perception more than anything else that tells of treatment success."

Born in 1955, Cuny has two daughters, the first born when she was sixteen. A detox client herself when she started working with youth groups on drug and alcohol prevention, Cuny says, "You have to start when they're ten, eleven, twelve, if you want to really do prevention."

Native American religion flourishes in Pine Ridge. Cuny explained that the Native American philosophy of healing emphasizes balancing the spiritual path, work and family.

"There have been more and more sweat lodges in the past ten years," she said. "We have medicine people and holy people. The medicine people know the roots and plants and where to find them and how to use them. The holy people know about spiritual things. Some medicine people can be holy," Cuny added. "You should talk to Wayne Weston. He's worked here before; now he's a drug and alcoholism counselor at the Red Cloud High School. Wayne has a presentation in which he compares Lakota philosophy with acupuncture philosophy."

In the fall of 1993, conversations with Weston and with Ila Red Owl suggested that acupuncture on the reservation had spread well beyond Project Recovery.

Weston was now director of the Employee Assistance Program (EAP) at the Oglala Sioux Tribal Public Safety Service. NADA-certified since 1987, Weston had become a NADA trainer, able to certify others; it is no longer necessary for NADA to send a trainer. Weston's acupuncture work, begun at Project Recovery, has included establishing and managing the Holistic Wellness Clinic, which existed for about four months until its planners ran out of building space and time. The clinic offered sweat lodge, meditation, acupuncture, and counseling.

Adult counselor and acupuncturist Ila Red Owl is a long-time Project Recovery staff member. Also NADA-certified in 1987, she says many of Weston's detox clients followed him when he moved to his present position. In addition to her counseling work, Red Owl sees about fifteen clients a month for a range of acupuncture treatment.

"Most are for arthritis or bone problems," she explains. "We still do detox, for weight loss and smoking. When we do body-needle treatment, we do detox treatment first." She mentioned treating a pregnant woman "for stress, to help her get through her evenings."

Weston says that interest in acupuncture is steadily increasing among law enforcement workers at Pine Ridge, but that the alcohol and drug people are not as enthusiastic. The Dade County program has attracted much interest among his colleagues. In the summer of 1993 Weston NADA-certified a pre-med student as well as the tribal police commissioner. The tribal chief prosecutor also wanted to be certified. Weston visited Lincoln that summer, taking some tribal people with him.

Weston enhances his acupuncture skills by sending away for literature and consulting with other acupuncturists across the country. His EAP clients—Public Safety Service employees—come for stress-relief treatment, as do school personnel. Many are skeptical, a factor which Weston appears to welcome. "I tell them, 'You don't have to believe, just see how you feel.'"

Weston continues to work with young people. He treats children aged eight to thirteen and diagnosed with Attention Deficit Hypertension Disorder (ADHD) with tiny glass beads—the kind used for Native American beadwork. Weston tapes the beads to ear points, especially Shen Men, "because the spirit is suppressed," and to Kidney and Liver points. The children respond so well that Weston gets two calls a week about ADHD. At high school athletic programs, he demonstrates, talks and treats, using acupuncture, moxa, cupping, Chinese masssage and acupressure as sports medicine therapies for adolescents. Sports medicine is an avenue by which to reach this age group for other problems.

Both Red Owl and Weston travel around the reservation to talk about and demonstrate acupuncture. Red Owl finds that people are more accepting of acupuncture now than they were when Project Recovery first used the method, and much less fearful about needles. The Project Recovery team continues to make presentations at sobriety campouts, where they find attentive audiences.

Thanks to the federal Office of Substance Abuse Prevention (OSAP), more money is reaching Native American reservations for prevention work, much of which helps teenagers.

Three times a year, twice in winter and once in spring, Ila Red Owl drives five hours to the Wellness Conference of another Sioux reservation—Eagle Butte.

"At Eagle Butte I treat from morning till evening, and then people want me to treat in the evening, but I'm treated out by then!"

Weston's acupuncture work has led to consultations and lectures at the Cheyenne River and Rosebud Sioux reservations and has recently brought inquiries from the Navajo reservation. His research in comparing acupuncture's medical philosophies with those of the Lakota is expanding in scope from a lecture (including one given at a NADA conference) into a book.

Some old people who know a great deal about traditional healing have heard of Weston's work, sought him out and given him further information. Traditional Sioux health-care knowledge was, for a while, dying out. Now this crosscultural medical analysis project has become a vehicle for preserving one aspect of local Native American history and culture.

9

"LINCOLN WEST"

"I've had two dreams in my life and I've seen them both come true. One was to set up a small independent chemical dependency clinic, which I did, at Somerville [Massachusetts]. The other was to mainstream acupuncture in a large, publicly funded chemical dependency and general medical clinic, and we've done that here." So says David Eisen, who directs a cluster of acupuncture-based programs and services in Portland, Oregon.

The heart of Eisen's domain is Portland Addictions Acupuncture Center. PAAC was established in 1987 at Hooper Foundation under the umbrella of Central City Concern, a private nonprofit organization whose main work had been to provide housing for homeless people, as well as transitional housing, and alcohol- and drug-free housing.

The deliberate plural "addictions" in PAAC's name is a detail for which Eisen takes credit only when pressed. PAAC treats 100 outpatients a day for detox and HIV conditions. Federal, state and county funds support the center. Medicaid clients receive bus passes. Eisen says, "I'm proud to say we consider ourselves the Lincoln of the West Coast."

New York–born Eisen's entire career to date has been in addiction treatment, most of it shaped by work that originated at Lincoln Detox. He is a NADA co-founder, an original board member and was elected vice-chair. He has been active at numerous NADA workshops, meetings and conferences.

After earning a master of social work degree at the University of Washington in St. Louis, Missouri, Eisen was hired as director of treatment at Archway House, a St. Louis residential addiction treatment facility with criminal justice clients. Archway used conventional methods, including talk therapy.

He read about Lincoln in 1978, and went to New York to investigate its methods. It was a difficult period in Lincoln's history but the work impressed Eisen, who came to work closely with Smith.

Eventually Eisen enrolled in the New England School of Acupuncture (NESA) near Boston, which at that time offered a two-year program. Acupuncture has drawn many Americans into career changes, but for Eisen it was more of a course-correction than a change of goal to acquire acupuncture skills so soon after embarking on his career. As for many others, working with chemical-dependency acupuncture at Lincoln was a transformational experience.

While at NESA Eisen continued to work with Smith in grassroots community-health organizing, which involved "sleeping on people's floors and paying expenses out of our own pockets," he recalls. He graduated in 1982 and set up Somerville Acupuncture Center, which continues to treat chemically dependent clients.

Eisen's speech to a judges' conference in Portland, Oregon, led to consultation work there. Eventually he was invited to practice in Portland.

Eisen is direct and practical when he talks about the development of his work in Oregon.

"At Hooper Foundation we got in as a pilot demonstration project, and we had eight months to put something together. In a sobering station we did some acupuncture and it was very ineffective—people were too sedated; it was blocking the acupuncture. We were in the drunk tank, but that was a small part of the population. When I came on I gave the drunk tank two weeks, and we nixed it. But in the fifty-four-bed [residential] unit upstairs, we really started seeing [acupuncture] work. We knew from our out-patient experience in Boston and New York that it would.

"Hooper had been operating for ten years before I came along. It was a nurse-run county detox program. These nurses were lord and ruler over a fifty-four-bed subacute medical facility. There were five of us and nine nurses. They had total control of the situation. It took nine months with weekly staff meetings to crack some smiles. There's just so far you can push, so you had to be very yin with it," he recalls, alluding to the yin-yang equation.

Slowly but surely the patient-seizure rate went down. Before acupuncture, nurses had to cope with five to ten seizures a month. In the four years after acupuncture was initiated, they noted six seizures in all. The nurses that re-alized their own stress level and burnout rate also declined, and patients needed less medication. Records show that after acupuncture patients' detox completion rate rose from 53 percent to 92 percent.

In 1991 the program was four years old. It had gone through a budget crisis with Oregon's new Measure Five limiting property tax, which is a major source of program funding. The acupuncture program was one of the newest around, and the structure of Measure Five cut into it deeply. The nurses told Eisen they would quit if the acupuncture program was cut.

Hooper's detox inpatients, picked up off the street, in-clude late-stage alcoholics with jaundice, hepatitis and cir-rhosis as well as a variety of other addicts. Most are dehydrated, some are vomiting blood and many show signs of imminent seizure.

PAAC's clients are addicted to many legal and illegal substances and combinations thereof: crack, heroin, speedballs (heroin mixed with cocaine), alcohol, metham-phetamine, Valium, Xanax, Tylenol 3 and codeine. Ranging in age from fourteen to seventy, most clients are between twenty and forty. Sixty percent are non-Hispanic white, 25 percent are black, 10 percent are Latino, and 5 percent are Native American. A few Asians come to PAAC for general medical acupuncture. PAAC also treats outpatients for detox and HIV-positive conditions.

Hospital emergency rooms, social welfare agencies, and probation and parole authorities refer clients to PAAC. A community mental health agency refers patients who are mentally ill as well as chemically dependent. PAAC also treats people who just walk in.

Because an addicted person is easily deflected from seeking treatment, PAAC sets up no barriers, and imposes no economic, psycho-social or medical conditions on the potential client. A walk-in gets a medical screening and within a half-hour is in the program getting treatment. Urine testing begins in the first week, after four or five treatments.

PAAC is a non-disease-specific clinic. Chemically dependent people sit next to people with HIV disease, who sit next to children with asthma, who sit next to older people with arthritis. A community clinic, it reflects the area's diversity, with black, white, Latino, Chinese and Japanese clients all receiving acupuncture in the room together.

Pregnant women and children of crack-using mothers also take detox treatment at PAAC. Practitioners tape small seeds to infants' ear-points, and recommend precise massage of these points. (See chapter twelve.) "Crack babies come along all right until they're about four," Eisen says. "Then they start to exhibit some real dysfunctional problems. At four years they become more sensitive, less innocent. You can needle children starting about the ages of four to six. Developmental and cognitive changes vary in children born exposed to drugs."

Five years after PAAC was established, Eisen was overseeing a network of programs and services. Some are acupuncture-based; others have an acupuncture component. In addition to Hooper and PAAC, with a combined daily census of 150, a program for pregnant substance abusers and infants at Emanuel Hospital sees ten to fifteen clients per day. A mental health program serves three to thirty dual-diagnosed people per day. A criminal justice program for people referred by probation and parole officers is at another site. Three residential treatment facilities run by other agencies provide acupuncture with counseling, or acupuncture alone. The HIV-positive program, with thirty to fifty clients, treats with acupuncture and herbs.

In October 1991 Oregon passed a law requiring that methadone maintenance be provided only *after* acupuncture treatment and counseling have proven ineffective.

"Now they're beginning to put some teeth into that," Eisen says. "Methadone is coming under fire here. There is a very high level of crossover addiction to alcohol and cocaine in methadone clients. We are reducing the positive urinalyses on the crossovers."

As in other NADA-based centers, PAAC clients who slip or drop out are welcome to return and frequently they do. It is impossible to overemphasize the fact that addiction is a relapsing disease. There is an amorphous quality to working with the unpredictable and elusive personality so characteristic of addicts.

Chemically dependent people are elusive on many levels, which is probably why so many conventional treatment methods adopt a tie-down, constrain, put-in-boxes, punitive approach which in effect says: harness an addict to social norms firmly enough and long enough and he'll straighten up and fly right. This puritanical approach has not been notably successful.

This does not mean, however, that PAAC is lax in its own overall approach. An effective program cannot mirror its clientele's ambivalent feelings and vagueness. Chemically dependent clients *do* look for "facts"—the comfort of a valid position on which to base an attitude. A client needs to know that she or he is actually doing some identifiable thing.

Everybody who comes into Eisen's programs signs a treatment contract. Goals and objectives and methods of reaching them are established. For instance, the contract might read: "Goal: to maintain clean and sober. Methodology: go to AA meetings five times a week; see your counselor once a week; have clean urines consistently for ten weeks. Goal: reduction in craving, depression, dope dreams. Methodology: have acupuncture daily for three weeks."

PAAC's definition of long-term treatment success is four consecutive clean-and-sober months, maintenance of an independent living situation and a balanced recovery. Official mileposts for client followups are four, six and twelve months from completion of treatment. PAAC receives a good deal of self-reporting on progress.

Eisen believes that the future of Chinese medicine in this country lies in exposure and its availability to as many people as possible. Especially in chemical dependency, he contends, there's no option but to do acupuncture.

PAAC not only serves clients, but also furthers acupuncture education. Third-year students at Oregon College of Oriental Medicine, where Eisen is on staff, work at the clinic on regular rotation, gaining experience in public-health acupuncture including the care of HIV-positive patients. They work under the direct supervision of nine different acupuncturists who are full-time staff members. (Oregon does not allow people with limited training to perform chemical-dependency acupuncture.)

In addition to his involvement with PAAC and related programs, Eisen treated inmates once a week in the local county jail until funding for that program was cut because of Measure Five.

Eisen's 1992 speech to colleges in Miami on treating HIV disease with Chinese medicine addressed an increasingly prominent aspect of public-health acupuncture and gave a mini-overview of the relationship between acupuncture and AIDS.

"Mary McCabe and I were among the first to treat people with HIV disease in Boston. Seven years ago when we started, people were literally coming to us and then dying within two to four weeks. They had full-blown cases of what was then called HTLV III disease. They were in vanquished yin and vanquished yang separation stage," he said, using traditional Chinese medicine terms describing nearly totally depleted vitality. "Even at that point the incredible power of acupuncture alone to help that passage from the physical plane to the next plane was evident. How important it was that people could be made more comfortable during the dying process. We have an incredible tool at our disposal with acupuncture.

"As time went on people were coming to us less sick. We were able to intervene at an earlier stage, so that we could increase the quality of life. We could look at normalization and stabilization of T-cell ratios. Hematocrits (a measurement of the relative amounts of plasma and corpuscles in blood) in red blood cells and white blood cells elevated and maintained. Cytomegalovirus and retinopathy and neuropathy started to ameliorate, often in conjunction with allopathic medicine.

"We're not in this alone, nor should we pretend to look at this as a cure. It is not. It's another medical intervention, but it's very powerful. Chinese medicine in general has a lot to offer people with HIV disease ranging from asymptomatic to full-blown AIDS. Acupuncture has an incredibly strong effect on relieving stress and anxiety. Tons of research show us the relationship between the immune system and stress and anxiety. Acupuncture offers us a very strong tool to affect that relationship.

"At PAAC it's not about 'doctor-patient,' it's about people working together. I don't know how we differentiate among factors which bear on increasing immune function, and quality of life, and

decreasing potentiation of opportunistic infection.
But wc do know that the model works.

"We have a saying in the field that silence
equals death. We need to speak out. We need to let
people know that this is a medical intervention
which, if done appropriately after proper diagnosis,
if done with the proper care, is an incredibly cost-
efficient tool to help people. If we don't tell them,"
Eisen went on, "people die. The same way we have
been telling the community for years that acupuncture works extremely well for chemical dependency.

"It's a little more dramatic in this culture now
with HIV disease. But you're not going to get AIDS
from treating people with AIDS. You're not going to
lose your practice by treating people with AIDS.
People are not going to shun you. The only thing
that's probably going to happen is your practice will
increase. And you'll be doing a better service."

10

PLAGUE WITHIN A PLAGUE—AIDS

No drug treatment center is untouched by HIV disease. Gay or straight, female or male, many addicts whom criminal justice and social service agencies refer for drug treatment are HIV-positive. Some women are HIV-positive addicts and mothers. Some children are born drug-affected and HIV-positive. NADA's involvement with treating HIV disease sprang directly from work with addicted people.

Because AIDS is a totally impoverishing disease, most AIDS patients seek treatment in public-health settings. Many American acupuncturists originally worked with AIDS at Lincoln or at addiction treatment centers that emulate it. HIV-positive clients—even those completely uninvolved with drugs—are by now routine fixtures in such centers. Modern plagues are intertwined. No place is very far from another anymore, so maladies spread across continents. Like bubonic plague, leprosy, malaria, sleeping sickness and syphilis, AIDS has pervasive human, economic and social consequences.

In the winter of 1979–1980, some homosexual men in San Francisco and New York City became very sick with clusters of symptoms not normally seen as precursors to fatal illness. Yet many of these patients died. Initially scientists referred to the syndrome as Gay Related Immune Deficiency (GRID). In late 1981 the same phenomenon was reported among intravenous-drug users. Gay men and IV-drug users are neither mutually exclusive populations nor necessarily identical ones. A February 1982 *Wall Street Journal* article stated that "a few early cases involved heterosexual drug users," and a Centers for Disease Control (CDC) task force on the new disease suggested that, with 251 verified cases, of whom 99 had died, the disease might be more prevalent than official statistics showed. The task force suggested that milder cases would not be reported. It was noted that IV-drug users with AIDS typically died of pneumocystis carinii pneumonia. A street junkie who barely made it to the city hospital emergency room in an advanced stage of pneumonia was unlikely to be considered the bearer of a strange malady.

Intravenous-drug users were notoriously apt to pass along disease by sharing hypodermic needles. Unprotected sexual intercourse would transmit it to non-drug-using partners.

By late 1982, with cases identified in women and additional heterosexual men, the disease was renamed Acquired Immune Deficiency Syndrome (AIDS). In late 1993 CDC statistics showed 339,250 reported AIDS cases over the preceding twelve years. In late 1994 CDC data indicated that IV-drug users make up one-third of AIDS cases in the United States.

Addicts at Lincoln's acupuncture clinic received general medical acupuncture when appropriate. From time to time clients appeared with unknown complaints. Later, when these complaints could be matched with the newly identified disease, clinicians realized that Lincoln's Acupuncture Clinic was treating AIDS before the disease had that name.

Experience accumulated to show that acupuncture for HIV-positive patients relieved general symptoms including weakness and fatigue, fevers, night sweats, diarrhea and swollen lymph glands. San Francisco Chinese herbal medicine expert Angela Shen, OMD, frequently consulted with Lincoln staffers and provided specific herbal formulas for people with AIDS. Historically Lincoln's method of treating HIV-positive clients was closely linked to its method of treating addicts. Lincoln Acupuncture Clinic treated 200 AIDS patients from 1982 to 1987.

As more public-health settings adopted acupuncture and independent free clinics sprang up, acupuncture treatment of HIV disease expanded. By the mid-1980s there was a movement to establish clinics based on patient demand and on clients' active collaboration. Private-practice acupuncturists—many of whom had trained at Lincoln—and other health-care professionals contributed regular treatment hours. Such clinics appeared in several states. An Illinois practitioner said in 1987, "Our state doesn't officially allow us to practice acupuncture, but who's going to bust us for treating AIDS?"

People diagnosed with AIDS pick their way through a minefield of pharmaceutical possibilities, drug costs and side-effects. Medications interact, adversely or beneficially. Some affect bone marrow so drastically that blood transfusion is required. Others produce digestive distress. Buffering agents can ease this but patients often must dose themselves at carefully spaced intervals, sandwiching the buffering agents between portions of medication whose action these agents can inhibit. Trying to regulate these variables is like trying to isolate each fragment of a swirling kaleidoscope.

Reports appear of some product that has mixed results on a small group of patients in Europe. Something else is still undergoing clinical trials, etc., etc. The HIV-positive population, for whom health-care self-education has necessarily become an obsession, keeps searching for effective medication that has no destructive side effects. This, and hope for a cure, motivate underground buyers' groups.

"I'm trying to stay as healthy as possible until they find a vaccine. Of course I know some people who've committed suicide. Who wants to linger in a hospital? I've made an agreement with a friend—we'll help each other out," confides an HIV-positive man in his mid-30s.

Chinese medicine diagnosis includes observation of tongue and pulse, and to a Chinese medical practitioner even an asymptomatic HIV-positive patient reveals a physiology that is already disturbed. A person not yet actively ill with AIDS may have a general malaise, a sense of not being quite right. At this stage it is possible to take supportive action such as changes in way of life, attention to nutrition, exercise and therapeutic group work in addition to acupuncture and herbs. Chinese medicine sees the body, mind and emotions as aspects of one package, all of which interact with each other.

Whatever the malady, traditional Chinese medicine's underlying principles are consistent: strengthen the patient by balancing her or his energy and thereby encourage the body's self-healing powers. Treatment aims to relieve stress and anxiety, strengthen blood-building organ systems and bolster the respiratory system, thus enhancing vitality. Herbal formulas for general tonic, immune system enhancement and anti-viral action have been used with good effect.

Acupuncturists treating people with AIDS collaborate with the patient, striving to prolong a decent quality of life by adjusting treatment in quick response to changing conditions. As a general rule, American acupuncturists and herbalists treat HIV-positive patients who also receive Western-medicine pharmaceuticals. To some degree AIDS has spawned a kind of ecumenical medicine. The process is by no means a full collaboration between Western and Chinese medicine; but as more MDs see more patients doing well with combined modalities, they become more tolerant.

Gay Men's Health Crisis (GMHC), which opened in New York City in 1981, was originally a support and information hotline for people with AIDS. The organization's three-fold purpose is education, advocacy and direct services to clients. Ninety percent of its funding comes from donations.

By 1992 GMHC had grown into a substantial community center whose 5,000 enrolled clients qualified for intake by having a medical diagnosis of AIDS/ARC (AIDS Related Complex). Despite its name, GMHC also serves women and publishes information addressing them specifically.

Among client services are four weekly acupuncture sessions, each given by a different volunteer practitioner. After securing permission from clients a GMHC official designated one session as most suitable for observation. "That's the best one for you to watch. It has to do with the way the acupuncturist works. In the others, the men are in their underwear, but this one has a different style." The acupuncturist was Dr. Michael Smith.

Acupuncture came to GMHC after a speech Smith gave at an Actors' Fund event. Someone who worked for recreation services at GMHC invited him over. "There were 30 people in a small room, and I said, 'Do you want a talk about acupuncture?' Silence. 'Do you want a demonstration of acupuncture?' Silence. 'Do you want me to treat you?' " Heads nodded; he treated. And he has continued to do so since September 1989.

Treatment frequency is a basic consideration with new acupuncture patients. Usually a patient is seen fairly often at the outset, then at greater intervals. Weekly treatment might not be the best possible schedule, but it was all that circumstances allowed here. Most GMHC clients, although treated only once a week, do not have recurrence of the fatigue symptom.

During two sessions, twenty-one men generously agree to discuss their treatment. Most of them have very clear opinions about acupuncture.

Fatigue and depression, standard early chronic problems for HIV-positive people, have such a tight reciprocal relationship it is difficult to say which triggers the other. All the men mention relief of the fatigue/depression symptom. Some commonly expressed opinions: "Regular medicine doesn't really have anything for us," one says. "It's all a crapshoot, but at least acupuncture and herbs aren't doing anything bad to my system," says another. "My doctor saw me trying to stop smoking and drinking and eat just the right foods and said 'you can't spend all your time being a perfect person.' "

Five or six men say they tell their doctor they are receiving acupuncture, but one does not because he feels the doctor would just be negative about it. Some are taking low-dosage AZT (Azidothymidine, 100 milligrams per tablet) three times a day.

T.J.*—a shaven-headed man over six feet tall in his early twenties—has had acupuncture for two years. He was taking low-dose AZT three times a day for two-and-a half years, but dropped it five months ago. "I didn't feel any different after I quit AZT. And I feel fine now," T.J. declares.

Not surprisingly, physical fitness is important to these patients. Most either do physically demanding work or go to a gym regularly. In this they resemble many in their generation; but in a room full of robust young men in treatment for an overwhelmingly frightening disease, working out has importance beyond muscle-definition.

With a few exceptions, the men are in their mid-thirties to mid-forties. Ethnic origins are evident only in the two Chinese and three black men. One man appears elderly. A client's wife reads the newspaper at a lounge table just outside the treatment area.

Several agree to talk while needles are inserted in the ear-points, but not after the other needles are in. One man states crisply that he will talk before or after treatment but absolutely not during.

Two clients for whom this is the second session follow

---

*Unless otherwise stated, patients are identified by first names which have been changed to protect privacy.

the routine: take an alcohol pad from the table, swab your ears and find a seat; for some, unbutton your shirt, remove your shoes and socks and roll up your trousers.

Smith reads pulses, examines tongues and makes one round inserting ear needles. He returns to the clients in order, swabs other points and treats according to need at foot, ankle, calf, hand, wrist and arm points. He treats a few at upper back points and several at a point on the head.

Ben is thirty-six. With his thick brown hair, moustache and heavily muscled frame, he appears forbidding. Of Italian background, he lives on Staten Island. He says he's had plenty of experience with needles, and really didn't feel anything at his first acupuncture session.

"You're a tough man," someone observes.

A big warm smile lights up Ben's somber face. "That's the image I try to present, but . . ." He shrugs. Ben goes to college, studying to become a Certified Alcoholism Counselor (CAC). He'll take more courses at Rutgers during the summer, if he's okay. No longer employed, he volunteers with an AIDS group on Staten Island.

Tom was diagnosed HIV-positive in 1988. He speaks with bursts of engaging humor. He has been receiving acupuncture for six months and reads all he can about Chinese herbal medicine. Tom is able to work at interior construction four to five hours a day without fatigue. He looks at the silent man beside him. "Jordan—I call him my coach—puts the vitamins list and dosage schedule on the kitchen door, so I won't forget."

Jordan had muscular dystrophy before he was diagnosed HIV-positive. He sits with trousers rolled awaiting the second stage of treatment. A plastic leg-brace stands in one shoe.

Lorenzo, diagnosed in 1988, can still work a half-day shift with the city sanitation department. "But I don't take lunch or breaks, which is how I can keep on working."

Lorenzo's Sicilian grandmother preferred traditional remedies to antibiotics, so acupuncture doesn't seem strange or threatening to him. A block-letter motto marched across the back of his baseball jacket: OUR LADY OF AGONY. "It belonged to a friend who died recently." He grins. "I went to a Catholic school."

Dan is amused to be told he looks about forty.

"I'm fifty-three—you've made my day," he laughs.

Born of Chinese parents in Hong Kong, Dan looks like a weightlifter. Despite his background, acupuncture was never part of his life before he was diagnosed HIV-positive about four years ago. He finds acupuncture relaxing as well as energizing, and manages without fatigue to work full-time for a government agency. Dan also takes Chinese herbal medicine—not only for AIDS, but also for colds and flu.

Harold went for a while to a licensed acupuncturist, but then his insurance company stopped paying. Then he went to an MD-acupuncturist until the insurance company found out that the physician was treating with acupuncture and again stopped paying. Which is why he comes to GMHC.

Lucky is twenty-eight and slender, with olive skin and lively black eyes. He was diagnosed about six months ago. He says acupuncture is "okay but one day I fainted. Dr. Smith said I turned white. He'd put a lot of needles up here on my back, for the liver, and he said what happened is my liver really reacted. Then I told him I had a history of hepatitis." Lucky is going to school, studying art history and French.

This is Jud's ninth treatment—he hasn't missed any for several months. By himself, Jud is renovating an apartment into which he must move in two weeks.

"I feel about the same as I did a couple of months ago. But my life is in turmoil. It's the deadline. I notice, when I leave here, I'm so relaxed. And it lasts through the evening, and the next day and into the night. I could get another treatment in the middle of the week, but it just isn't convenient to take time from the apartment."

Andrew is having his fourth treatment. He took AZT but could not tolerate it. He works full time in a middle-management position supervising twelve people in a publishing house.

Thirty-four-year-old Frank has ruddy-brown, wavy, short hair, sherry-colored eyes and a strong sense of humor. This is his third acupuncture treatment. He was diagnosed HIV-positive in October 1991.

"I'd been tested two years before, and was negative. And I hadn't done anything to get it, in between."

He thought he had a cold, which turned out to be pneumonia. He was not short of breath but when his chest felt heavy he went to his doctor, who put him in the hospital, where he remained for three weeks on intravenous antibiotics and steroids. When he left the hospital, he began taking low-dose AZT five times a day. It cost $200 a month. He saw his doctor for pentamidine aerosol every two weeks. That cost $250 a month.

Frank couldn't tolerate AZT. "My hematocrit [percentage of red cells in the blood] had gone to 11 percent; the usual is 40 percent. Six weeks ago I needed a transfusion. One time, three units of blood, cost $800.

"Then I switched doctors. The new doctor is on the Board of Infectious Diseases at NYU Medical Center. He stopped the pentamidine and I started Bactrim [a sulfa drug] tablets. No more office visits for aerosol, so it was a lot cheaper, about four dollars a month. I stopped AZT and switched to DDI [another anti-viral drug] and today I got the news that my hematocrit is normal, but my T-cells have dropped."

Told that his patient receives acupuncture, Frank's doctor said he doesn't know enough to have an opinion about it but has heard it is useful for some people.

Clients sit for 45 minutes with needles inserted. Some meditate. Two read newspapers. Experienced patients remove their own needles, and help each other with those that are hard to reach. Carefully they deposit used needles through a hole in the top of a large red box. As the last patient finishes, the box is taken to an office where it is locked away. When full, it goes to a company which disposes of hazardous waste.

According to Smith things have changed from several years ago: now you see many different symptoms, perhaps as a consequence of patients taking various medications, perhaps for unknown reasons. People don't always want to tell what medication they're taking.

On April 29, 1992, the New York City Council's Committee on Health heard doctors' and acupuncturists' testimony on a resolution proposed to the New York State legislature. Resolution #110 calls for health-care underwriters to provide policies that reimburse for acupuncture services rendered by licensed acupuncturists.

Frederick Nesetril (his real name), a GMHC client, submitted testimony in support of resolution #110. Here are excerpts.

"I am a 44-year-old gay man, who has lived and worked in New York City since 1969. I have been a New York City employee at the Human Resources Administration since 1990.

"I have been HIV-positive since 1979.* Since 1984, although I have remained HIV-positive with a diagnosis of AIDS according to current CDC standards I have not resorted to traditional Western medical treatments for my HIV-related conditions. (I took one Western drug, acyclovir, for two weeks, the first time I came down with herpes zoster in 1984.) Instead, I chose acupuncture, herbs, homeopathies, vitamins, and a diet that ranged from a healthy balance with no milk and few meats to a standard (less-than-healthy) 'American' menu. Although my T-4 cells

---

*Nesetril's blood was frozen in 1979 by the New York Blood Center and tested later in 1984, as a part of Dr. Cladd E. Stevens' HIV follow-up study to the group she had tested and studied for Hepatitis B.

dropped from 400 to below 200 range, since 1984 I have not had any major opportunistic infections.

"The fact that I have never been hospitalized or suffered a major opportunistic infection since 1984 is no small feat. . . .

"I have never been unemployed due to HIV-related illness. Since I began my employment with the City of New York Human Resources Administration two years ago, I have taken no more than five days of sick leave. . . .

"Acupuncture costs less than traditional Western treatments currently available to HIV-infected people. For what it cost to see a Western medical doctor and treat my herpes zoster, I could have had several acupuncture treatments, which would have not only prevented the zoster, but would have generally treated my condition (immune suppression). Western medicine is symptom specific. . . . Acupuncture is holistic and treats the whole body. For people who have immune dysfunctions, it is less costly to treat the system than the symptom. . . ."

Ilka Tanya Payan—actress, immigration lawyer and former New York City human rights commissioner—loved a man who used drugs, infected her with HIV and subsequently died of AIDS. Payan was diagnosed HIV-positive in 1986, and says her doctors told her she would die in five years. At first only close family members and a few friends knew of her condition, which progressed to AIDS. She feared losing theater and television work so she kept quiet about her HIV status.

In October 1993, she publicly disclosed her condition. In December 1993, she spoke at a United Nations World AIDS Day forum. Like Frederick Nesetril, she has avoided drug medication. For a number of years Payan received acupuncture and herbs from a Chinese practitioner, whose physician-associate read Payan's medical charts.

During that time Payan regularly visited her native Dominican Republic where most of her family live. While there she maintained an acupuncture regimen at Dr. Frank Canelo's Devanand Clinic.

In 1988, remembering actor friends who had died of AIDS, Payan became an advocate for people with HIV.

Since October 1993, she has been a client at Gouverneur Hospital's Dr. Daniel Leicht Assessment Clinic (for HIV-positive people), which referred her to Gouverneur's acupuncture clinic. Initially she received ten daily ear-acupuncture treatments, according to the NADA protocol, for stress reduction. "It really changed my thinking," she says, "I developed a different attitude; I don't have anxiety anymore." She receives ear-acupuncture at Gouverneur three times a week. One of these sessions also includes full-body acupuncture. Because Payan is currently unemployed her Gouverneur treatments are free.

Many more cases like these have been documented by acupuncturists and herbalists such as San Francisco's Misha Cohen and Chicago's Mary Kay Ryan and Arthur Shattuck. A national conference is now held annually on the use of traditional Chinese medicine in treating AIDS, attracting several hundred practitioners.

11

"A Hundred and Twenty Babies"

San Francisco's Bayview–Hunters Point Acupuncture Clinic lies south of the city in an African-American community on the western edge of San Francisco Bay. Hunters Point is the site of a defunct naval shipyard, whose structures, still Navy-owned, are leased to the city. Along the shore, empty streets lined with rows of vacant sheds embody desolation, until you notice signs that some are occupied by small businesses, manufacturing plants and social welfare agencies. Inland are a number of one- and two-story attached houses— "projects," California-style.

A converted shipyard building houses the acupuncture clinic. Inside, the large pleasant sunlit room holds a screened-off treatment table and about thirty-two chairs which stand in rows alternately facing each other and back-to-back. Two more tables occupy a smaller adjacent room.

Next to a corner window a bright cloth-draped table bears a couple of eagle feathers and assorted amulets. Two years ago a Yoruba woman performed a ceremony for the clinic at this altar, to which people still bring significant objects. Across the room hangs a large, framed print in which a nude black man, prone atop a yellow wall, reaches down toward the upstretched hand of another black man.

In the spring of 1991, two and a half years after Bayview–Hunters Point Acupuncture Clinic opened, staff includes four acupuncturists working with a clerk and fourteen counselors. Thirty-five to fifty clients a day present a range of conditions. One-third of the treatment is general medical acupuncture. Families with or without addiction problems, are treated here, as are stroke victims and people with AIDS. Pediatric clients include babies with AIDS and drug-exposed infants and children Other youthful clients have no drug exposure at all. Some children have problems at school; others do not. In the clinic's experience, school problems do not necessarily correlate with drug-exposure history.

In addition to treating, Bayview's licensed acupuncturists supervise interns from local acupuncture schools. Treatment is available seven mornings a week at Bayview and five afternoons at nearby Alice Griffith Medical Clinic.

Everyone enrolled in Bayview's crack-cocaine program must come for acupuncture, but this treatment is not the only service the clinic offers. Bayview is the heart of many activities, including clients' birthday celebrations and various expressions of African-American spirituality. The Friday "After Hours" program, exclusively for acupuncture clinic clients, emphasizes coping skills—how to get a GED (General Equivalency Diploma) or a scholarship and how to acquire the tools to control one's life and expand choices. To maintain recovery people need encouragement to make productive choices. Educational and women's support groups proliferate at Bayview, and men's groups were started because the men felt left out. Also available are Narcotics Anonymous, Cocaine Anonymous, groups focusing on parenting, beginning recovery and advanced recovery.

One April morning in 1991, observers from Santa Clara County's Bureau of Alcohol Services came from the southern end of San Francisco Bay to tour Bayview. One of them had heard a lecture that Bayview's acupuncture clinic director Patricia Keenan delivered two months before at NADA's Santa Barbara conference.

Women, children and a few men received treatment unperturbed as the Santa Clara people looked on. Three visitors accepted the invitation to experience treatment. Each visitor took a copy of the clinic's information sheet.

Clients in adjacent chairs compared sensations and reactions with their guests.

"See, it's no big thing," said one, immediately putting a stranger at ease.

"Makes you feel relaxed," says another.

A mother walked past pushing a child in a stroller. There was a small square of tape on the child's ear. Another young mother displayed her infant: he wore two squares of tape on his small translucent ear.

"He's smiling," observed a visitor.

"Yeah, but I think that smile is gas," the sixteen-year-old mother replied with maternal authority.

Tape on the ear is a visible sign that these children are acupuncture patients.

Trained in China, Patricia Keenan is known in American acupuncture for developing the treatment of drug-exposed babies and children. "When I first saw babies needled in China, I was freaked!" she remembers.

Following a three-and-a-half-year stint as Bayview's director of acupuncture services, Keenan is now a consultant on acupuncture and chemical dependency treatment. She held a variety of community-based jobs before committing herself to acupuncture. She was a nurse's aide in a U.S. public-health hospital program for alcoholics and addicts in San Francisco and was a volunteer at Lincoln Detox for six months.

After a California acupuncturist treated her for sciatic problems, Keenan inquired about acupuncture schools, and soon began classes at San Francisco College of Acupuncture. She knew she wanted to be an acupuncturist, but instead of entering private practice was determined to work in community health.

Keenan comes from a working-class family of seven, five of whom had long-term addictions—to heroin, cocaine and alcohol. Her father was an alcoholic. The question of quality family medical care has always been an issue.

After two years of acupuncture college Keenan spent three months studying acupuncture in Nanjing, China. She returned to California, where she passed the Acupuncture Board examination. During the next eight months she worked in a number of volunteer and paid part-time jobs: with mentally ill homeless people, at a detox center in San Francisco's notorious Tenderloin, and at Quan Yin Clinic under Misha Cohen. (A pioneer in using Chinese medicine to treat AIDS, Cohen worked at Lincoln Detox early in her acupuncture career.) Finally Keenan was hired by Bayview–Hunters Point Foundation for Community Improvement, a twenty-year-old African-American foundation.

Bayview had been using methadone for fifteen years when its staffers set up a three-year research project on heroin. The project used acupuncture.

"We started out as a drug clinic, but three weeks into the research project we were treating anybody in the community. That's how we came to treat babies," Keenan remembers. The clinic became a primary health-care facility for the entire Bayview—Hunters Point community.

Keenan, who was Bay Area NADA coordinator for five years, sees community health as a foundation for social justice. "A community health clinic, has the capacity to treat whoever walks in the door—old, young, teenagers, addicts, pregnant women, etc.—and to be a role model of a healthy community. And to help people apply the guiding principles of the model to the community itself."

Keenan is a strong advocate for the babies who became her specialty. She challenges superficial media portrayals of addiction which present it as a black, inner-city problem while virtually ignoring white addicts and those who can afford private health care.

"A baby's symptoms can sometimes be drug-related. I see drug-exposed babies from the moment of birth to three, four and five years of age," Keenan reports. "But in private hospitals, unless the baby is in writhing withdrawal it is not tested for drugs. So what may seem to be irritability in an infant, may in fact be withdrawal."

Keenan deplores the popular press' use of the term "crack babies." She is concerned that children labeled as such will be plagued throughout their school years by the self-fulfilling prediction of failure. They must be diagnosed and treated in order to be educated and grow into adults who contribute to society, she insists. Treating drug-exposed babies from the time they're born gives them a chance to fight the negative label.

Keenan notes that some affected babies are actually suffering from methadone withdrawal rather than from street drugs. "Methadone withdrawal is painful for children, but in this country," Keenan explains, "clinicians prefer to put pregnant heroin or crack addicts on methadone, and the baby is born addicted to methadone."

She concludes that the media has exaggerated drugs' permanent damage to babies but the less-sensationalized fetal alcohol syndrome (FAS) is clearly dangerous. "A lot of babies who have been exposed to drugs are fine. A small percentage have permanent brain damage. Babies who've been exposed to alcohol run a high risk of brain damage. Most of the women who have extensively damaged babies were abused during pregnancy, and used multiple drugs.

"None of our children have become emotionally disturbed. But they say if you don't see that problem at six months old, you'll see it at two years. So we're continuing to watch."

Outreach, treatment and education are inextricably

linked at Bayview Acupuncture Clinic. Staffers often give talks and acupuncture demonstrations throughout the community—in schools, for public-health nurses, in daycare centers and for grandparents' groups.

To reduce her audiences' fear, Keenan needles herself while the children watch, and always she allows somebody to needle her. "I only let them needle me in LI 11 [a point on the forearm], the least painful on me." Many patients come because of the children who participated in these demonstrations.

Keenan has been in practice since 1987 but she does not profess to be an expert in Chinese medicine. She *is,* however, an authority on babies who have been exposed to drugs because she developed the protocol for treating them with acupuncture. First she picks up an infant and holds it for a period of time, feeling its energy and muscle tone, determining where it's tight, asking if it is a comfortable baby. With the holistic approach that characterizes Chinese medicine, she stresses the importance of having a sense of who the baby is, and of the mother's relationship with the baby.

"If the mom is very uncomfortable about the baby, it means she's frightened, it's her first child or she feels that she's not going to be an adequate mother."

She examines the color of the face and the expression in the eyes for an alert spirit—a quality often absent in drug-affected babies. If the problem is beyond her professional scope she refers the young patient to another practitioner. For example, Keenan sends babies with ear infections to a Western doctor, because babies can go deaf very easily and these infections respond well to antibiotics.

Just as infants exhibit rapid developmental changes, most of their health problems also change rapidly. When babies

---

*Acupuncture needles *can* cause pain, but it generally is fleeting. Inexpert insertion may be painful.

are two or three days old it is generally not necessary to needle them. Energy can be moved by acupressure with a finger or by *tuina*—Chinese massage—and by pressing ear-points.

For ear-point pressure on infants and children, Bayview uses an herbal seed, *semen vicaria,* which Keenan learned about in China. It doesn't irritate the baby's skin. About the size of a mustard seed, the semen vicaria, stuck to a piece of adhesive tape about half an inch square, is placed so that the seed itself lies on the ear-point and will stimulate it when the tape is pressed gently. The seed is used mechanically, not pharmacologically.

The mother learns to press each seed ten times, three times a day. Keenan says that in Chinese medicine the intention is sometimes three-quarters of the treatment. She tells the mothers, when pressing the seeds, to say aloud to their babies, "You are going to be a well-developed child; you are healthy; you are growing; you will make a contribution to this society; I love you." Keenan emphasizes the importance of applying pressure *gently* because many people who feel guilty when their babies are sick live in the land of more-is-better.

Participating in the drug-affected baby's treatment is also beneficial because it allows the mother a central role in the healing process, which assuages her guilt and induces her to stay in treatment herself, because she wants her baby treated.

Points Keenan uses for treating drug-affected babies include Shen Men in the triangular fossa; Kidney, high on the concha; Stomach, in the midregion of the concha; Spleen, also in the concha but lower and farther away from the face; Brain Stem, a little below the helix-tragic notch; and Brain Spot, adjacent to Brain Stem but closer to the face. Not all points are used at one treatment: points are selected according to the patient's condition.

Keenan uses Shen Men to calm the person and clear the mind. Stomach and Spleen are used often. The other point used consistently on babies is the Kidney point, because this point is responsible for maturation and for brain development. Kidney deficiency is present in a number of children Keenan encounters, which she speculates is because this African-American community has limited access to medical care.

Practical clinical experience affected development of this pediatric protocol. Keenan originally used Lung, the point next to a baby's ear canal, but a seed taped at one infant's point got lost and couldn't be found. Although the baby never showed signs of a foreign object in the ear canal, to reduce future risk Keenan determined to find another point to use instead of Lung.

Referring to a Chinese ear-acupuncture manual, Keenan noted that the point Brain Stem (farther from the ear canal than Lung) was described as effective in conditions like trembling, and arching—bending the body backwards, head toward soles. And an adjacent point, Brain Spot, was identified as "good for hypnotic stare," an accurate description of the gaze seen in many drug-exposed infants.

"We started trying those two points, and it worked immediately," she says.

For the first months the baby is seen every four days if the mother is compliant. After that, treatment is once a week; and in the eighth, ninth or tenth months it changes to once every two weeks as long as the baby progresses well. When the baby has a cold or stomach problems the clinic also provides its primary health care.

Marcus was one month old. His grandmother, who worked at the clinic, said Marcus was a lovely child. The baby never cried. "She put him in my arms," Keenan reports, "so I walked around in the foundation showing off the baby. The baby never moved: he felt like a board." This was a phenomenon Keenan remembered seeing in institutionalized children who were severely disabled mentally, emotionally or physically.

"I needled Shen Men and handed the baby back to the grandmother, and the baby went 'Ah-h-hh.' It was the most remarkable thing. Then I needled Lung. The next day the grandmother said, 'Marcus cried from nine to eleven last night.' I said, 'Good! The baby hasn't cried for a month, he's got a lot of catching up to do.' By the time he reached twenty months he had become a normal, healthy, well-adapted child with no tightening of the muscles.

Children who tremble have seeds applied, and they stop. Babies used to staying up all night at seven days of age have a seed applied at Shen Men and they sleep. "These are consistent reactions," Keenan says.

Keenan is careful not to overtreat a baby, and to take specific conditions into account. Many babies born exposed to drugs are premature and at two months may weigh only five pounds. They often have neurological difficulties. When they're asleep, their hearts sometimes can stop. Consequently, such a child is equipped with a heart monitor whose beeping awakens the mother and alerts her to shake the baby. This caused concern about using the Shen Men point, because it is calming. "Do we want the baby sleeping more?" Keenan asked. "You'd have to shake the baby all night long. I'm a very cautious person when it comes to infants, so I said, 'Let's leave out Shen Men in these premature babies; let's only use Kidney.' In three weeks' time every single baby's development was unbelievable."

Educating mothers, fathers and designated caregivers—who are often the babies' grandmothers and great-grandmothers—about acupuncture treatment is part of the job at Bayview. Keenan always explains what she is about to do, and shows how she's going to do it, including needling the baby.

There is constant reinforcement of the proper way to press ear-points. When babies have difficulty sleeping despite ear-point treatment, mothers are taught to administer a diluted form of Sleep Mix formula—a blend of camomile, catnip, hops, peppermint, skullcap and yarrow—It is the same tea the mothers receive. Mothers are also encouraged to use their own judgment, although given their addiction history, many feel insecure about doing so.

"We tell the moms they can take the seed off if the baby's uncomfortable for whatever reason. If the mom is uncomfortable, take it off. The mom should be the last word. If the mothers know that we trust them, they can trust us."

Ideally, when a diagnosis is made, all who care for the child are involved, because the mother may only see that child for an hour a day. Many great-grandmothers raise children and do it very well. "Sixty-five, with a baby six months old! We treat them for stress. They're very honest about what's happening to the baby. They're not the addict, so they don't feel they have to please you."

Addicts beginning to recover often change in ways their friends and families are not always ready to accept. Couples might have been walking around each other for years because one partner is deeply preoccupied with getting and using dope or drink, and is psychically absent even when physically present. With recovery, long-suppressed emotions surface and find expression. While adults have trouble coping with recovery's dynamic shifts, the phenomenon can be even more disturbing to older children, who are often as profoundly affected by their parents' recovery as by their addiction.

Because craving rules the addict's life, regaining control over that life is an important aspect of recovery, proof of progress in overcoming addiction. But the shadowy fear of slipping back into chaos can make such a person obsessive about control. The child of an addict who has done things pretty much his or her own way (and that covers a range of activities like never washing, sneaking a beer for breakfast, or skipping school), can be shocked by the sudden intrusion of responsible adult supervision.

One such child, Keenan says was angry with her mother for six months: "What do you mean by behaving like a mother," the youngster demanded. "I've been running this pretty good, and now you're taking over!"

Because of these problems, parents under treatment are asked to bring their children in on a regular basis, even if the children aren't being treated themselves. This way the children will understand that the parent is changing because something tangible and important is taking place in his or her life.

One hundred twenty drug-exposed babies had been

treated at Bayview-Hunters Point Acupuncture Clinic by April 1991. At the time Keenan emphasized that even so, "We're brand new. It's like the infancy stage of doing babies here."

12

WOMEN AND CHILDREN

Since medically supervised civilian drug-addiction treatment centers first opened in the mid-1960s, most clients have been men. Women junkies stayed in the background; generally their men supplied them with street drugs. Women were not a factor in considering program design.

Times changed faster than treatment: in the mid-1980s crack brought a galloping increase of women addicts. Now women constitute 50 percent of crack users, many of whom begin smoking the drug while pregnant. Treatment for pregnant addicts in conventional settings remained limited and rarely appropriate to their maternal requirements. Most women clients have children who accompany them, or who are in child welfare custody—either way, children motivate their mothers to succeed in treatment. But in group counseling sessions it has been difficult to focus on the needs of a few women while addressing the needs of the male majority.

As an addiction counselor explained, "A woman may be the only one here, and she feels alienated, and pressured by the men. The guys start to compete, showing off. It's hard to confront your own problems and to have to keep warding people off. Women get that in the street. Why come here and get it too?"

A women in treatment often faces the quandary of involvement with a man who doesn't buy into what she's doing for herself. It's hard to choose between a program and family members or lovers who sabotage the process of recovery. (The same mentality affects the dieting woman whose partner says, "You look fine to me.")

Addicted women, their children and their relationships are central to the domain of Nancy Smalls, LPN. Smalls is the director of Maternal Substance Abuse Services (MSAS), established in 1987 at Lincoln's Acupuncture Clinic. A Prenatal Clinic and nurse-midwife were added three years later.

The area around her ground-floor office bustles like a marketplace. Women clients' business with staff is interspersed with maternal concerns: "Take that out of your mouth, that's not candy!" "Could I have a Pampers for the baby?" "I need some condoms." A visitor must take care not to trip over a very short person temporarily detached from its mother.

For a couple of years, "The basement is not ready yet" summed up the frustration of an ever-receding horizon.

The six-week MSAS program begins with a ten-day cycle of detox and daily urine sampling. This can be repeated until counselor and client agree that the preponderance of negative urinalyses warrants moving on to the program's next phase—fewer acupuncture treatments per week. While crisis counseling is always available, at this stage of the program women must attend a Narcotics Anonymous meeting once a week, as well as a weekly women's group. Every clinic visit includes acupuncture and leaving a urine sample. (Many patients need a longer program, but agency, time and volume needs press for a short course.)

MSAS takes into account women's obligations outside the clinic. About 80 percent have been referred by the Child Welfare Administration. The program encompasses long-term treatment in order to show authorities that a mother has been drug-free long enough to regain custody.

More than 50 percent of court-referred clients—people who have not voluntarily sought treatment—show two months of drug-free urines in the program. Collaborative, not coercive, treatment style and record-keeping make it easy for lapsed clients to rejoin the program. Many clients return for further treatment after completion. "With the acupuncture, I know I won't pick up again," they say.

Recognizing that mothers of young children have housework to do and must struggle for time, MSAS consolidates program requirements into one block of time per visit, usually about two hours. (An underlying lesson of this arrangement is learning to be on time, a basic skill for future employment.)

Clients have ranged in age from twelve-year-olds to people in their fifties. Many are third-generation welfare mothers. People who have spent a lifetime dealing with welfare and related systems learn never to be anywhere on time because they have so much experience in arriving at an office and having to wait, seemingly forever.

Most women's groups cover practical topics such as safe sex, AIDS education and family planning. Clinicians clearly explain that having ten children by the age of thirty is not necessary. "I tell them you only want two or three children at the most because it is exceedingly expensive to raise these kids," says Smalls, herself the mother of six. "It's overwhelming. But I was a nurse, I had a job."

Women's group sessions are also psychologically educational and supportive. Ninety percent of MSAS clients have been abused—physically, sexually or both. Many are incest survivors. Smalls and her colleagues think the women's drug use might be a way of suppressing their feelings about such histories.

Much anecdotal evidence suggests that patients receiving general acupuncture for physical complaints report a sudden and profound release of emotional anguish during treatment. "Sometimes when you use acupuncture on a person who has been sexually abused as a child," relates Smalls, "the acupuncture opens up thinking channels, which means opening a Pandora's box. This person is going to think about stuff she hasn't thought about for twenty years."

In addition to these peak emotional events, group sessions focus on general indignities experienced by poor women of color—women who are deprived, depressed and degraded.

"With this program we try to re-educate, retrain, make these women think," says Smalls. "Your life doesn't have to be forever around welfare and begging and low self-esteem, this man beating you and you can't do anything. You do have some rights. We validate that this black or Hispanic person has a place in the world and didn't just come out from under a rock."

Not surprisingly, Smalls and her team, found that success in building self-esteem in their women clients created problems with male partners who resisted change. Some men would respond by beating the client and then coming to the program to complain.

MSAS formed a men's group, conducted by Jesse Morgan, partly to deal with many men's reactions to loss of control over their women, and partly because men felt left out.

Smalls claims to have found out that a man, regardless of color, thinks that wherever he lays his head and eats, he comes first. "They feel if they come home with fifty dollars and want to go to bed you're supposed to stop what you're doing and go right then, whether the kids are running around or it's high noon." The fact that participants openly express such attitudes in the men's group is impressive. "So we've got to retrain both sets of folks. The men begin to realize that it's okay to have some feelings; it's okay to cry, it's okay to touch somebody, have some emotion."

The basement was to house a daycare center, appropriate for infants to school-age children. This center would achieve several objectives: women's group sessions would run more smoothly without the distracting presence of children, and children would be better off in a place designed for them instead of tagging along while their mothers engaged in program activities. Also, hands-on parenting skills classes were urgently needed in order to break the ugly tradition that abused women are in turn apt to abuse their children.

The program's expansion lurched into existence over a three-year period. The basement leaked; and rats, as Smalls says with her characteristic irony, "were seriously coming in out of the weather." With Lincoln Hospital responsible for the building, necessary repairs to the physical structure were delayed or stalled, never quite meshing with timetables of grant awards and disbursement requirements. Furniture and equipment were stored.

Grant-approved specialists joined MSAS in a working/holding pattern: talented staff can't be hired at the last minute. For a while, lack of a basement telephone was a major obstacle. "How can I have a parenting skills class with little children and no telephone?" Smalls exclaimed.

In November 1992, the recently opened parenting skills center was gleaming new. An outsider couldn't help but share Smalls' triumph and delight when she opened the door to the twenty-four by forty-foot space.

Gwen Alford, nurse-practitioner and parenting skills specialist, is in charge of the unit. She explains that children are cared for here while mothers are in treatment, although some mothers prefer to keep babies with them while they receive acupuncture.

Alford conducts a tour of the center, which is open five hours a day. "It's everything you'd want if you were a little kid, isn't it?" she says. At one table, Alford's assistant Celeste May, an early childhood education specialist, holds an infant while his eighteen-month-old brother pushes crayons over paper.

Nothing here is makeshift or hand-me-down, but fresh and purposefully arranged, modeled on early childhood centers in any middle-class community. Toys are geared to creative play and to spark the imagination—no bulbous plastic wheeled vehicles. A wooden stove stands next to a cupboard with realistic plastic food. Child-height easels hold paints and plenty of paper. There is clay, and colored papers, and a bright carpet for adventurous crawling. Alford uncovers the sand-and-water table, saying she really had to fight to get it. "Why shouldn't these kids know what it's like to play with sand and water?"

In addition to rocking chairs and low, round tables with child-scale chairs, the furniture includes a playpen and four clear plastic hospital-issue cribs for newborns. Long bolsters, on a thick pad spacious enough for mothers to join in, form an exercise area for babies. Observing casual parent/child interaction reveals specific problems that staffers can address in parenting-skills classes.

Alford says some children are unaffected by maternal drug abuse, while effects on others show up over time. It became evident that some children lack normal fine-motor coordination: Alford describes a four-year-old boy who could not do the simplest peg-in-board games, even though his three-year-old sister was very good at them.

Although women are normally the prime caregivers, it is defeating to expect the mother to improve her parenting skills without involving the man she lives with, whether husband or boyfriend. He is part of the household and must be constructively involved. Men also have been victims of childhood abuse, and are equally apt to carry on the tradition. Therefore men's group clients participate with women in MSAS parenting-skills classes. As one man remarked, "I don't have to hit my kids any more, because I can talk to them."

Change in small children occurs rapidly. After parents

see how quickly their children become vibrant in the daycare room, they start wanting to keep the benefits going at home. Alford gave a class assignment in which students were to make a toy or learning device out of items in their homes. They were not allowed to buy any materials. One student painted the alphabet on a pillow in bright block letters; another brought to class a two-faced rag doll—one face was a girl's, the other a boy's; another student created a doll whose face was painted on a tea-strainer. The strainer's cloth-wrapped handle was its body; plastic forks were hands and spoons were feet. Another student's overstuffed cloth doll had "HUG ME" on her chest and is pillow-soft. A father built a tractor-trailer truck of corrugated cardboard. This precisely detailed working model measured nearly two feet long, in perfect proportion, with drinking straws for axles. A man living in a shelter soaked a washcloth with glue and molded it around a jingle-bell to make a ball for a baby's delighted mystification.

Since its inception, Lincoln's MSAS unit has increased and expanded its services. Midwife Lea Rizack's schedule has been doubled to two days a week. Following establishment of the prenatal clinic, a one-year study of pregnant patients showed higher birth weights—averaging seven pounds, six ounces—in infants whose mothers consistently attended the program and received acupuncture. Pregnant women who use crack cocaine tend to produce low birth weight infants—defined as under five pounds—who require hospitalization. Low birth weight is associated with respiratory problems, among other disorders; and also with a diminished fortitude which, although not measurable, is evident in the baby's response to the ordinary rough encounters of daily life.

Another common problem has less to do with the infant's objective condition than with the taint of being born drug-affected. Sometimes a doctor who is told that a child's mother is addicted lets that fact dominate a diagnosis. Thus, an internal congenital problem can be overlooked because an infant's reactions are attributed to maternal drug use.

The federal Office of Substance Abuse Prevention (OSAP) funded a project, sponsored by the New York State Department of Health, allowing MSAS to hire four peer counselors and their coordinator who also does counseling, crisis intervention and court advocacy. This new element is called the Sisters Program. "Sisters" trained in case management interview women, "hold their hands" during detox and make sure they go to court appointments. These helpers also accompany clients through the endless court proceedings to secure visitation rights. Sisters sometimes go with pregnant clients to the hospital when they deliver. The peer counselor component is significant not only for staff expansion, but also because most women completing the MSAS program have not had the chance to become counselors. The job is a solid step out of dependency into professional work.

Maternal Substance Abuse Services and the prenatal clinic see over 120 clients a day, about half of Lincoln's total census. The facility's effect on its primary clients has wide consequences. By actual count one parenting-skills class of fourteen adults touched the lives of seventy-five children.

13

THE NONADVERSARIAL COURT

"The President of the United States says to build more jails, throw you junkies in and let you rot," the judge says, looking around the courtroom. "Why did you quit on me?" he asks, peering over his glasses at the slender young man standing before the bench, who replies, "I didn't quit. I just didn't go."

"Been with us about one and a half years," says the judge, reading a computer printout.

"Punch it up, and you'll see nothing but cleans," the young man states boldly.

"Your fees for your treatment were paid by the guy before you," the judge reminds him. "You pay for the next guy. I suggest you pay *something* weekly. Between graduating and sealing the records is six weeks. I expect you to make some payments." (Drug Court clients are assessed fees on an income-based sliding scale. Fees range from $500 to $2,500, for annual incomes of $5,000 to $50,000 or more.) The judge flashes a small smile. "Recommended for graduation," he says. The young man straightens up, grins and nods agreement.

A 1950s movie starring Spencer Tracy as the judge? No. We are in Miami, the crack cocaine capital of the United States, in the spring of 1992. The scene is Drug Court—officially, Section 51, Criminal Division, Dade County, Eleventh Judicial Circuit of Florida—Judge Stanley M. Goldstein presiding.

Section 51 was established effective June 19, 1989. That year, Dade County had a major problem. Eighty-seven percent of persons arrested had cocaine on them. At the same time, an accumulation of drug-related convictions in the 1980s had resulted in overpopulated prisons. The county faced a $1,000-per-day fine because of jail overcrowding.

Under the former system, drug offenders not charged with violent crimes were shifted from court to probation to treatment. The system lost track of many in the process. Goldstein says that then, in the first two weeks of counseling, assessors lost another percentage before they even figured out what the offender's problem really was. Only about 6 percent of those arrested on drug offenses in the old system went into recovery. The majority kept going in and out of jail.

Now Goldstein can assign most offenders immediately to outpatient acupuncture/counselling sites. But at his discretion clients can be assigned to one of two residential sites (parts) where acupuncture detoxification is provided. One of these sites is for men, one for women—short stays only. "Long-term residential treatment is garbage. You learn to live without cocaine within the program, but you don't learn to live without cocaine outside the program," the judge insists.

This court, which handles eighty to one hundred cases per day, is the first in this country to conduct business without an adversary system. Cooperation among prosecutor, public defender and judge characterizes Drug Court proceedings—the purpose is to get addicts into treatment instead of into jail. Law enforcement, public-health and social-welfare agencies all operate under a kind of Olympic truce in their customary turf war. Their remarkable collaboration benefits addicts as well as Florida taxpayers.

The man in Goldstein's court, busted in September 1991 for possession of cocaine, volunteered for the court's Deferred Drug Program (DDP), a Diversion and Treatment Program (DATP) for substance abusers. In his year and a half as an outpatient, the recovering addict progressed from the thirty-day intensive Phase One, in which he received daily acupuncture treatment and counseling until, with seven consecutive clean urines recorded, he qualified for Phase Two. In Phase Two he received acupuncture and counseling three times a week and appeared before Judge Goldstein, who evaluated his progress before promoting him to Phase Three, during which he received monthly acupuncture treatment and continued to give urine samples. Throughout this, he managed to hang on to his day-labor job. With nothing but clean urinalyses for several months—and thus drug free—he stopped attending the program.

Drug Court is held in what looks like a standard courtroom, but a morning's observation shows how profoundly it differs from traditional courts. It lacks the virulent hostility and air of bitter hopelessness prevailing on both sides of the law in ordinary courtrooms. Drug Court officials are polite to defendants and DATP clients, and rather protective of them, too.

The noticeable absence of lawyerly histrionics differs markedly from other courts. In Drug Court, as in acupuncture, the focus is on the client. From the defendant's first contact with the system, great care is taken to keep him or her on board and progressing toward the goal of becoming—or rebecoming—a productive member of society.

The jury box holds defendants, most of whom are brought straight from jail. Some look dazed. Most appear shabby and undernourished. All qualify for Drug Court because they have no record of violent crime and are first-time cocaine offenders.

About thirty spectator seats accommodate women and

men who look like any multi-ethnic group of city people on their way to work. These DATP participants must appear at stipulated intervals to tell Judge Goldstein how they're doing. They enter and leave by the public door, like any other citizens; but over several months' time in the program they hear again and again Judge Goldstein's pep talks to new people, which include the refrain, "This is not easy. It's the hardest thing you'll ever do in your life." Observing the newcomers, who reflect their own sorry condition when they entered the program, encourages them to continue.

After arrest, defendants who qualify for the program are kept in cells separate from those who don't. Here, Pre-Trial Services personnel explain the program to them. Inducement to enter the program rather than gamble on release from the overcrowded jail system includes treatment for addiction; and upon successful completion of the program, a cleared record.

About 90 percent volunteer immediately for the program; the rest have a chance to change their minds in the course of the day.

Both volunteers and non-volunteers go to Drug Court for bond hearing the following weekday morning. In Drug Court volunteers are assigned to the program. Counselors report to the court and relevant agencies on the defendant's progress every sixty days. Non-volunteers receive an explanation of alternatives—basically, this entails going through the regular court process and being sentenced to as many as two and a half years if found guilty.

"To those who are here for the first time," Judge Goldstein says, "I'm your bonding magistrate. I determine what the bond will be." He then reads the Miranda rights, and emphatically cautions defendants against self-incrimination, because if their case ever has to go to court, what they say here could be used against them. When several cases have been heard, a woman with no visible teeth begins to explain her circumstances, and the judge interrupts to repeat the warning. He does so in the same even tone each time a defendant makes this error.

Judge Goldstein works with a smoothly functioning team which includes both prosecutor and public defender, court officers and a bailiff, many of whom speak both Spanish and English equally well. Interpreters promptly assist clients who speak only Spanish, or whose English is not fluent.

The public defender, Hugh Rodham (brother of First Lady Hillary Rodham Clinton), is a vital contributor to the design and successful conduct of this unusual court. Without the public defender's understanding that treatment benefits his clients, he would normally try to get them off with credit for time served, and back on the street as quickly as possible.

Because close attention to detail is essential to keeping the DATP package together, the program has very strong reporting requirements. A participant with three absences from the clinic is automatically reported to Pre-Trial Services or to a probation officer, and to both the state attorney and the public defender.

Excuses for missing an appearance are not lightly tolerated. For example, if a participant fails to show up in court simply because the notice was mailed to a former address, he or she might still be dismissed from the program. Judge Goldstein makes it clear that participants must notify not only the counselor, but also the clerk of any change of address. It is their responsibility to do so.

A middle-aged man's record shows that his weekend urines are dirty, but the samples are clean the rest of the time. "Whoever you're meeting," Judge Goldstein directs him, "take her to the program with you." The man begins to object. "It won't cost you extra," the judge insists. "The dirties, that's when you're meeting with somebody, whoever she is. Take her with you."

One woman is a recovering drug addict not living at public expense. She has school-age children and would like to attend the program after she finishes work at 7 A.M. Her shift starts at 11 P.M. She works near the program site, but the program's afternoon session ends hours before she travels to this part of Miami on her way to work. She could tend to her household and get a decent stretch of sleep if she didn't have to make a second round-trip by bus to comply with her present program schedule. Judge Goldstein orders, "Fix it so she goes in the morning."

The snarled cord connecting drug-addicted women and children resists untangling. One strand is straightened out, then another kink appears and more knots form. A defeated-looking woman in her forties is here to tell the judge that her daughter has run away with a boyfriend and abandoned the program. Left with her daughter's child, the mother says sourly, "Programs don't work."

Judge Goldstein reviews the daughter's recent record: thirteen out of fourteen urines are clean; her behavior in the program had been good. Based on the mother's testimony, he orders that a warrant be issued. But he makes it clear that if the young woman appears of her own volition he will do everything he can for her. If she is picked up on the warrant, "she's in trouble." The judge seems to be more on the side of the absent daughter than her mother is. It's not unusual—parental fortitude wears out, professionals keep on going.

A young woman, whose long blonde hair frames a round face, is here to explain a charge of Failure to Appear. In the program—during her second trimester of pregnancy—she gave dirty urines three days in a row. Her boyfriend, with pompadoured hair and nailhead-studded denim suit, stands in the well of the court holding their three-month-old baby. She is pregnant again. The prosecutor suggests assigning the baby to State of Florida Health and Rehabilitative Services (HRS). "I want my baby," she whines. "And if I gotta go to residential, my boyfriend can take care of him."

Judge Goldstein declares that the baby will go to HRS. "I'm going to see that you get residential treatment for two weeks, with daily counseling. Then you'll have a fighting chance to make it on the street." Buford looks relieved.

One of the young men looks to be seventeen, but is older. He has been doing well in the program. He asks if a recent misdemeanor bust for public disorder and verbal assault on a police officer will cause trouble for him. Judge Goldstein tells him to go upstairs and find out his case number. As the young man heads for the door, the judge sends the bailiff with him in case there's a problem up there. When this offender and the bailiff return half an hour later, the judge orders the misdemeanor charge allocated to this court so that it stays within the package of the man's DDP case.

Preventing small incidents like this from blooming into large ones underlies Drug Court philosophy. Gonzalez could easily slip deeper into trouble if he stood in the wrong line, asked the wrong clerk for the case number, became discouraged and left without reporting back to Drug Court. Then if for some reason he was picked up and a prior misdemeanor showed in his files, he could be held and arraigned in a different court and consequently miss his acupuncture and counseling sessions. All too easily his progress could be nullified.

In a system that provides every opportunity for offenders to slip and risk arrest, Drug Court—paying scrupulous attention to detail—hand-carries participants into compliance until they make enough progress to live responsibly.

Another defendant, a thin man with thick glasses, has been caught with "goods" on him. Judge and lawyers consult in low voices. Judge Goldstein explains gravely, "The stuff you have here is not cocaine." The defendant looks baffled. "What you have in this bag is pure sunbaked dog doo-doo." He looks around the courtroom and informs everybody, "It sits on the street and the Florida sun bakes it white and the dealers scrape off some of that white and mix it with the cocaine to extend it. But there's no cocaine at all in this." The judge relates another drug-dealer trick: they take the white crust that forms on a car battery—solid battery acid—and add it to cocaine. "You don't always know what you're getting from the dealers," the judge concludes. This defendant is dismissed.

A diabetic DATP participant is absent. The judge uses this gap in the calendar to tell his audience, "For a diabetic, using cocaine is like putting a gun to your head and playing Russian roulette."

After the judge has variously praised, lectured and encouraged them, the DATP participants leave. Many are headed for their jobs.

Today's defendants have all chosen the program. Some, as the judge tells them, look as if they could use a good night's sleep. These defendants will begin short-term residential treatment; others will go directly to a program site to start outpatient treatment.

After the calendar has been completed, Judge Goldstein relates some history to courtroom visitors.

Goldstein, whose street-cop humor is clearly appreciated by those who appear before him, is a former criminal-defense lawyer. He believes in encouragement, not in threats. In Drug Court he deals with all kinds of people—millionaires, the homeless, doctors, lawyers, and the unemployed.

While he talks to the visitors, court staff wraps up the morning session's business. Today's defendants are being assembled for their trip to residential and outpatient treatment. Each shambling woman has one handcuff around a bony wrist, the other attaching her to a long chain. On the men's chain a defendant carefully and politely holds the door open for the court officer bringing up the rear, who equally politely thanks him. One woman rolls her eyes and laughs silently. You get the feeling that court officers and defendants alike think the chain-and-cuff technique silly, but how else to get a pack of spaced-out or withdrawing people from one location to the next? The scene is like that of urban teachers shepherding young school children to the park with each child grasping the guiderope.

Linked to the Drug Court process is a Substance Abuse Aftercare program associated with Miami-Dade County Community College and occupying two locations. Aftercare—available but not compulsory—provides oversight, education, vocational training and job placement to graduates of DATP's third phase. As Judge Herbert Klein wrote in a 1990 letter to then-Federal Narcotics Commissioner William Bennett, "Our purpose is to provide [addicts] with the tools to become productive members of society, as well as the tools to stay drug-free. The cost of this [aftercare] program is $350 per client."

Dade County's NADA-based program has wide implications for unclogging the U.S. criminal-justice system. It's not just the prisons that are overcrowded with low-level users and dealers, but also court calendars. The "war on drugs" produces huge criminal statistics, but no place to treat addicts. Outpatients receiving acupuncture treatment keep coming back to the program, even if they slip from time to time. "We're on the right track," Judge Goldstein remarked.

Another Dade County population receiving acupuncture treatment for addiction resides in the county jail, known as the Stockade.

Dade County's Stockade is a sprawl of low, cream-colored buildings surrounding a grassy area. In odd corners tropical plants, locked behind black Spanish-style grillework, rustle in the 7 A.M. breeze.

The resemblance to a tropical village ends when you see the twelve-foot-high metal fences topped by concertina rolls of razor ribbon. The routine is like that of any jail, a start-and-stop herding of approved visitors who sign in, wait to be counted, then shuffle through one gate which must shut behind them before the one ahead can open. Visitors pass a building over whose doorway Times Gothic letters proclaim, "Freedom Chapel."

In a grassy open area clusters of men exercise and lift weights. Some do laundry. Others who had breakfast at 4 A.M. line up for lunch.

Treatment takes place in a "temporary housing" build-ing. Two acupuncturists treat seventy-five to eighty people during the 6:30 to 10:30 A.M. session. These prisoners have plea bargained, accepting a short sentence with mandatory treatment as an alternative to a five- to seven- year sen-tence. In the thirty days of Phase One they have a mini-mum of fifteen acupuncture sessions, and attend three therapy groups a day. In Phase Two, which lasts sixty days, they have individual and group therapy every other day and continue with acupuncture as needed.

Each participant arriving for treatment walks in, selects a card, and picks up a service-log form and tray with alco-hol swabs and needles. Then he swabs his ears.

Following treatment, which proceeds as calmly as in other NADA-based clinics—no jailhouse atmosphere here—the card with the acupuncturist's notations is returned, along with the form and the tray. The acupuncturist counts the needles before the prisoner leaves the room.

The Stockade was the scene of the first public acupunc-ture demonstration in a U.S. criminal-justice setting. Mae Bryant, Director of Dade County's Office of Rehabilitative Services, remembers that event.

When Smith made his first visit there, she says, some of the prisoners were taken out of the regular in-jail treatment program and led into the room.

"With all the media there, we were in the back of the room, holding our breath," Bryant recalls, "and in maybe eight, ten minutes he and Carlos Alvarez [Coordinator of Lincoln Acupuncture Clinic's Criminal Justice Project] treated about fifteen people. One guy was adamant about how he was not going to do it; he didn't need this! And of course all the cameras went directly to him. He was the last person they showed on the news, fast asleep with his needles in his ears."

Bryant visited Lincoln at Judge Klein's instigation, and was involved in planning the Dade County programs from the beginning. She directs a 350-person staff, fifty of whom treat patients in both the diversion program and the jail program. As for choosing people to work in the acupuncture treatment program, she explains, "That staff got selected because we knew we were doing something different. We looked for people who had flexibility, who were not tied to the old treatment methodology and who we thought could form rapport with clients quickly. We developed a one-week training session with Janet Konefal, giving them complete acupuncture information."

Dade County hired Dr. Janet Konefal—acupuncturist, associate professor at the University of Miami School of Medicine and director of its masters in public health program—to develop the acupuncture programs.

Florida does not permit counselors to give chemical-dependency acupuncture unless they are licensed acupuncturists. From the outset, most of the fully trained acupuncturists hired for the drug treatment program were Asian. Acupuncture easily crosses cultural barriers that might exist between Asian practitioners and clients from many different ethnic groups.

Defendants involved in the jail program called Treatment Alternative to Street Crime (TASC) are sentenced to 364 days or less—although most get 364 days. When they have successfully completed the program, they can get early release, with the remainder of the sentence on probation. During that time they attend the Aftercare program.

The first thirty days in TASC are spent in total lockdown, with nothing to do but focus on treatment. The next ninety days are more flexible. Work might be assigned, but in addition to the job at least six hours a day of treatment-related activities are required—activities such as NA or AA meetings, group therapy or "homework" to do in the cell.

Bryant's experience makes her confident about the strength of acupuncture's ability to facilitate drug treatment. "We don't require acupuncture. It's voluntary. And we don't sell it. It sells itself. It's the people who tell each other, 'I feel better.' If you can come into our program and give me seventeen clean urines in twelve days without needling, then you don't have to go [to acupuncture]", she asserts. "But the problem is, you *can't* do that without needling. So you either find yourself staying in Phase One longer, or deciding, maybe I better go over there and see what this is about."

The Stockade's custodial personnel, Bryant says, have come to see that the inmates' acupuncture treatment benefits them as well. "They don't have to deal with as many confrontations. Inmates are generally in better moods, so it's made their work easier," she asserts.

When Bryant talks, it all sounds reasonable, logical and easy. But establishing the Dade County programs required a great deal of attention to detail, legwork and coordination among the district attorney's office, the courts, the public defender's office, the jails and treatment people.

Miami's Drug Court has continued to develop: acupuncture treatment is available in the Turner Guilford Knight (TGK) facility to which Judge Goldstein, at his discretion, sends selected clients for brief residential treatment. TGK now has ninety-six beds for men and forty-eight for women.

Dade County's Drug Court shows what can be done when innovation is ordered from the top, and those at the top are powerfully committed to backing up those who implement the change.

14

THE BANKS
ARE MADE OF MARBLE

In a forlorn area of New York's South Bronx an imposing triangular building points to the subway overpass shading Westchester Avenue. Carved stone letters above a no-longer-used entrance at the building's apex spell out its former identity: MANUFACTURERS HANOVER TRUST. A painted sign above a side entrance says "El Río."

A bank being used to house social welfare work calls to mind Les Rice's song that was popularized by Pete Seeger:

> But the banks are made of marble,
> with a guard at every door,
> and the vaults are stuffed with silver,
> that the farmer sweated for . . .
> I've seen my brothers working,
> throughout this mighty land,
> I prayed we'd get together,
> and together make a stand.
> Then we'd own those banks of marble,
> with a guard at every door.
> And we'd share those vaults of silver,
> that we have sweated for.

Dade County's Diversion and Treatment Program was a direct response to an overwhelming situation in the local criminal-justice system—the sheer numbers of people arrested. Dade County risked financial loss as surely as drug offenders risk incarceration.

El Río was similarly formed to deflect jailbound, drug-affected people from clogged institutions. Housed in a former bank building, it opened in July 1990, with a treatment program modeled on that of Lincoln. Guided from the start by a former Lincoln staffmember, El Río, like Oregon's PAAC, embodies NADA's acupuncture detox and recovery-maintenance methods.

El Río was originally designed with a fairly narrow mandate: to treat crack-involved young people who were at risk of going to jail. But with acupuncture's holistic approach to health care, the center grew rapidly into a supermarket of services for a wider range of drug-involved clients.

In May 1991, El Río's Alternative to Incarceration (ATI) program for drug-involved residents of Upper Manhattan and The Bronx was nearly a year old. Funded by New York state and city agencies as well as by private foundations the program was conceived as acupuncture-based intensive daycare—9 A.M. to 3 P.M.—for addicted people who would otherwise be imprisoned for at least six months. It was officially termed "a drug-free ambulatory substance abuse program." El Río has always operated under the umbrella of Osborne Treatment Services, an affiliate of the Osborne Association, a nongovernmental, nonprofit New York criminal-justice agency established in 1933.

El Río's clients—defendants, probationers and parolees— were defined as being at least fourteen years old and using crack. They were referred by probation, parole, and several other ATI programs.

Clients attended a structured six-hour program five days a week. It included a nutritious breakfast and lunch that were flavorful and attractively presented, unlike most institutional fare. Clients received daily acupuncture-detoxification treatment. In aftercare—during recovery—treatment was given at greater intervals. Classes, cultural activities, Narcotics Anonymous meetings and counseling filled the schedule. Altogether the program entailed six months of intensive full-time day treatment followed by six months of aftercare.

Interior renovation of the triangular building created offices, a library, a small meeting room and an acupuncture room. Remnants of the building's previous incarnation included marble counters topped by bronze-grilled tellers' windows and ground-glass signs. The counters enclosed the former central banking floor, converted to a general-purpose open space with sofas and round tables for meals.

A guided tour led past the hulking bank vault, anchored in cement to bedrock, and chained open. This area now held a laundry room and a bathroom with a shower.

Some clients would arrive having slept in their clothes, without having washed or changed. The guide, named Reno, in charge of safety and fitness, ran down his no-nonsense approach to this problem:

"You're not in the land of the living dead. The counselors and the rest of us may have to put up with you, but you're putting yourself in a box just as if you went to prison", he pointed out. "So there's the washer and dryer, and there's the shower. Nobody says you have to use them; but you'll like yourself better if you do."

Having done time, done college, done Vietnam and done bodyguard work, Reno was a calm, genial, absolutely self-possessed man whose suggestions you would be inclined to follow.

The bank's basement was transformed into a spacious ceramics craftsroom—complete with firing kiln—and a kitchen with restaurant-quality stainless-steel equipment. A professional chef was in charge, assisted by a client preparing to graduate from the program.

At lunch with staff and clients one diner remarked, "I only been here a week, but it's funny, I used to smoke a pack a day and I noticed yesterday, it's a pack in three days. I don't know, maybe it's the acupuncture."

Davine Del Valle, NADA-certified in 1986, is the in-house program's assistant director. Animated and with a relaxed sense of humor, she talked about El Río's program, breaking away from time to time to resolve some difficulty requiring an immediate decision.

El Río's fourteen-member full-time staff included four administrators, some of whom were responsible for other Osborne Association programs; a fiscal officer and assistant; a general administrative assistant; five counselors; the chef and a maintenance engineer. Three part-timers taught classes once or twice a week in ceramics, *tai chi*, other exercises, writing and poetry. Some staff members are themselves in recovery, some are not.

Del Valle said, "We all have different backgrounds. And we have all kinds of traditions here—Hebrew, Christian, Islamic, people with a strong Native American belief system, Buddhists. And we have the twelve steps of NA."

In an acupuncture-based program, treatment is integral to the routine, not an optional extra. It is also standard practice to make acupuncture readily available to staff members. This is done as a proven stabilizing factor. Del Valle said that she regularly had one or two counselors present while she treated and called out names of points. Some counselors would soon go to Lincoln's Acupuncture Training Institute to be certified.

In addition to ear acupuncture for detox, some clients with severe health problems received general medical acupuncture from the licensed acupuncturists.

"If somebody has asthma and they're having a bad time with it, of course you're going to respond to it," Del Valle said. For example, flu-like symptoms sometimes occur during detox. In these cases the acupuncturist inserts extra needles at points that help counteract flu symptoms.

El Río's philosophy, Del Valle explained, is to support the recovery process, "not to slap people's hands and beat them down. They get enough of that."

Urine-test policy varies from one treatment center to another. Del Valle explained why El Río tested at random:

"Not only is daily urine testing costly and time-consuming, but it can undercut other priorities. But you must test, because of denial."

Behaving violently or getting high on the premises was cause for termination. However, clients who continued to use drugs were not necessarily dismissed. Del Valle expressed a concept similar to that of AA: Valid progress is made when a client admits to an addiction problem rather than continuing to deny it.

One program client, compliant, a lovable and good-hearted man, appeared like clockwork every day, without a problem. But he still used drugs, though not at El Río. From 9 A.M. to 3 P.M. he didn't get high, which reduced his intake, but he did not stop altogether. Potential disaster awaited him every time he left the bank. Finally, after months of denying his problem, he confessed that he needed residential treatment.

"From my perspective that was a success," said Del Valle. "Some people can only deal with going off drugs cold turkey. They just can't go from drugging to walking in our door. Others can."

El Río would refer clients who needed it for brief inpatient detox, after which they could return to the program.

El Río had very few women clients, and what few began the program often dropped out—a fact of great concern to the mostly female staff. Del Valle said they were trying to develop a track specifically for women's problems. She said that women sometimes brought their children to the weekly open NA meeting, but that the program had no scope for childcare. The open plan of the ground floor and basement common areas were not practical for children.

Staffers had recently submitted a proposal to the Department of Health outlining a track for pregnant addicts and their children. A monthly alumni group would enable those with day jobs to visit friends and staff in the evening, hold meetings, see films, enjoy some refreshments and feel like part of something—and to know that they didn't have to stay unwell to be a part of it. "In the twenty years I've been doing this kind of work I've noticed a lot of people don't get well because they don't want to lose the program," Del Valle commented. "They start regressing as soon as they're on their way out."

Several years into El Rio's existence, the bank's exterior remained as it was, but fewer men were hanging out on the street, and more private cars were parked at the curb. Change, physical and programmatic, is evident in the building's humming interior.

When the commercial tenant vacated the second floor in 1991, El Río took over that space along with a cluster of related Osborne Association programs.

Visitors can't walk up the old marble staircase until a polite but careful sentinel—whose blue shirt displays an Osborne Association patch—verifies the visitor's errand by telephoning the second-floor receptionist, who can look through the windowed door and see who is waiting to be buzzed in.

Surveillance cameras monitor the second-floor reception area with its blue-gray, wall-to-wall carpet and comfortable seating. Clients wait here to see counselors for individual sessions. Pale-coral-colored partitions separate this space from the offices that occupy the rest of the floor. The area retains a clean, bright, just-moved-into look.

A side table holds a wicker basket of brightly wrapped condoms. Coffee tables offer flyers advertising drop-in groups for women alcoholics, for lesbians with HIV/AIDS, for a Clean & Sober New Year's Eve Dance. Pamphlets in Spanish as well as English present useful, straightforward health information:

"WHEN YOU'RE WITHDRAWING YOU CAN'T THINK OF ANYTHING BUT GETTING YOUR DRUGS. BUT NOW YOU'VE GOT TO THINK TWICE: about AIDS, what it is, AIDS and drugs, AIDS and Sex, AIDS and your children."
"SAFE SEX IS A LESBIAN ISSUE."
"WHAT YOU NEED TO KNOW ABOUT TUBERCULOSIS."
"BROTHERS LOVING BROTHERS: safer sex for gay men."

Ana Oliveira, the Osborne Association's Director of Services, trained at Lincoln Acupuncture Clinic. She was head coordinator for several years, and responsible for staff training. She also taught the course in acupuncture for chemical dependency at the New England School of Acupuncture, near Boston. (She was succeeded by Terry Courtney.) She is on staff at Lincoln's Acupuncture Training Institute; and since 1989 has taught a course on addiction which is part of the Master's Program in Public Health at Hunter College. As a founding NADA board member, she undertakes regular speaking engagements, at which she performs with thought-provoking eloquence. In June 1992, she was elected NADA chairperson.

Oliveira came to El Río when the project was still on the drawing board—at that stage it was nothing more than a proposal that had been approved by the New York City Deputy Mayor's Office of Public Safety. When Oliveira joined the project as Program Director she and her associates modified the proposal and guided it from paper to reality, a process which involved renovating the building as well as planning programs.

Oliveira's promotion to Director of Services at Osborne in late 1991 initiated a six-month transitional phase beginning in January 1992, during which, she says, "We organically broke El Río down into pieces defined as services, and restructured into units of service. Now any service is available to any client."

This goes against standard social-work principles, in which clients are pigeonholed and populations are not mixed. (El Río still provides acupuncture-based substance abuse services, but the definition of its clients has changed: they no longer need to be jailbound.)

"The system outside identifies you and splits you, so outside they catch you, or they diagnose you, or they label you *one thing:* HIV-positive, or chemical dependent, or "problems with the law." But in here there's a true holistic approach, in the sense that the person is treated as a *whole* human being. And that goes for meals, subway tokens, substance abuse, recreation, HIV education and counseling."

In addition to El Río, Oliveira's domain now includes Living Well, a case management and service program for people who are HIV-positive or have AIDS; Assigned Counsel Alternative Advocacy Project (ACAAP), an Alternative to Incarceration program; Family Works, a parenting program for fathers at Sing Sing; and an educational program here at the former bank. Some services are new; some older ones have recently been modified.

"Osborne always had the Bureau of Vocational Placement—primarily about finding jobs, and now part of a larger service which is Educational and Vocational, job placement being one piece of it," Oliviera explains.

New in the past year are Health Services and Referral and Advocacy for Treatment (RAFT)—"the raft that runs on the river," says Oliveira, referring to the fact that El Río means "the river" in Spanish. "And there's La Fuente—[the Fountain]—a high-tolerance program that uses acupuncture detox. It also provides crisis intervention, meals, referrals, and HIV education in all forms for people who are chronically failing. La Fuente offers an incentive to come into treatment."

All services at the former bank building are prioritized according to the principle that the *client, not the funding source,* is the focus. These services look to the clients' needs. Since very hierarchical pyramid programs don't work over time, El Río was divided into smaller units that have one coordinator and a small staff, a strategy that affords clients more personal contact, interaction and responsibility.

Further improvements have been made in the building. Expanded health services have taken over several ground-floor rooms formerly used for offices. Computerized urine-testing equipment has been installed, allowing daily urinalyses for substance abusing clients. The program monitors and tests urine daily, and over 82 percent of these samples come out clean—a very high percentage. The daily test covers cocaine, heroin, marijuana, and Valium. Every two weeks a test is given covering nine drugs. No one has complained about the change in procedure from the former random testing.

Medical exams are given twice a week. (Women clients are referred to other facilities for gynecological services.) The screening exam is El Río's first health-care contact with clients, and it takes place early in the intake process. Staff members are screened for TB every six months. "See, up here?" Oliveira points to the examining room ceiling. "This is vented to the outside." [A precaution against accumulation of airborne TB bacteria.]

An adjacent room, with plants on the divider walls, contains two acupuncture treatment tables. It is sectioned off by an attractive wooden cupboard holding large jars of Chinese medicinal herbs.

This storehouse of Chinese herbs is a *formulary*—a collection of individual herbs in natural form, portions of which can be blended into various formulas according to a patient's condition. Generally these mixtures are brewed into a drink.

The former meeting room and library is now the carpeted detox-acupuncture treatment room. Panels of printed African kente-cloth decorate the walls and relaxation music plays softly. An alcove has been made from the long-boarded-up doorway that was the building's main entrance in its banking days. Door-height fanciful metal grillework is backed by glass bricks through which sunlight casts water-pattern shadows onto large, live green plants. There was no money for decoration, but by allocating a little here and a little there, it was done for less than $100. Aesthetics are not a funding priority in clinical settings, but Oliveira insists that her clients be treated in a civilized, attractive ambience. "Just because they are poor," she asks, "why should it be ugly?"

Health care expanded in the program's overall revision. Carla Wilson, RN, L. Ac., left her private acupuncture practice in Austin, Texas—where she also worked at the Austin Immune Health Clinic and taught at the University of Texas Nursing School—to become El Río's Health Services Coordinator in February 1992.

When she started, acupuncture detox was provided, and a physician was on duty—sometimes one day a week, often not at all. Wilson launched a project that involved just giving chronically sick people vitamin C and basic Chinese herbal medications. Also, she addressed acute conditions like colds, flu, viral and upper respiratory infections.

The herbal medications Wilson uses are traditional formulas in patent form, modified to deal with specific conditions and produced by herbal pharmacological companies in China, the United States and elsewhere. Yin Chiao, for example, a 2,000-year-old herbal formula now available in tablets is a common remedy for the onset of colds and flu symptoms. It is used for three days, after which if the condition goes deeper (when, for instance, a cough produces yellow phlegm, and depending on *how* yellow) another medication might be administered. This is usually one containing the herb isatis (*Isatis oblongata*) which has very strong antiviral, anti-inflammatory, and anti-infectious properties. For a condition which still does not improve by the end of the day, a Western antibiotic might be used.

Demand for basic services quickly produced too much work for one person, so Yolanda Castro, L.Ac., was taken on as health assistant and plans were made for additional staff.

Another physician visits two days a week. Health Services provides medical screening and TB screening. According to the protocol all incoming clients must first take
a TB test, the Mantoux skin test.

Many clients coming from parole, probation and work
release appear without medical records, which can take
weeks to arrive. With the late 1990s' increase in regular
tuberculosis and proliferation of medication-resistant strains,
TB testing protects both clients and staff. In addition, Carla
Wilson says, "The Living Well [HIV-positive] clients moved
here in April [1992]. We have this ultrasensitive population, so we have to consider the implications of TB."

HIV-positive clients are treated with acupuncture and
Chinese herbal formulas, alone or in conjunction with Western medication—mostly AZT or Bactrim, occasionally
pentamidine—through the Health Services clinic called El
Río de la Vida (The River of Life). El Río de la Vida is
specifically for people coping with a compromised immune
system or with some chronic illness, not only for HIV-positive individuals. El Río de la Vida clients all take herbs and
see primary-care physicians. Blood testing is part of the
Living Well program. "El Río de la Vida is successful and
growing," Wilson states. "We're seeing predictable results,
which I recognize from my work in the Austin Immune
Health Clinic."

Wilson's administrative work and treatment, like that of
many public-health acupuncturists, is inextricably involved
with teaching. Detox acupuncture, provided five days a
week, takes place in the context of other health services
work. Wilson gives counselors a basic understanding of
Chinese medicine and how it fits into the facility, of the use
of herbs and other supplements, and the importance of
diet. Her teaching provides a solid foundation to those
counselors who go to Lincoln's ATI for NADA training.

El Río's inherent possibilities progressed from concept
to reality over a period of eighteen months. Daycare hours

have doubled—the program is now open twelve hours a day, and three daily meals are served. The chef now has two assistants who are acquiring marketable skills. There is a structured alumni group. Whereas clients formerly had to be jailbound and were limited to the specific service for which they were enrolled, they no longer need criminal justice sanctions, and every service is available to every client.

From 900 to 1,000 clients pass through the bank annually. Cost per client for the first six months of enrollment is annualized at $7,000; for the second, less intensive six months, per client cost is annualized at $3,000—roughly $10,000 per client retained in treatment. El Río began as the only acupuncture-based service in the building. Now, acupuncture is part of overall health services, including the Wednesday-night community clinic. Acupuncture, always available to staff, affects the general climate of work.

Opened in October 1993, and a now likely model for other localities, New York City's Midtown Community Court hears misdemeanor charges—so-called "quality-of-life" crimes—such as shoplifting, soliciting prostitutes, stealing rides on public transportation, and unlicensed vending— for which penalties do not exceed a year in jail. This court usually sentences defendants to minimal fines and several days' community service instead of jail. (So far the community court's clients have shown 80-percent compliance with community service assignment whereas generally people sentenced to community service simply fail to turn up.) The judge urges them to take advantage of classes in English as a Second Language, as well as other educational and vocational services, all of which are provided on the sixth floor of the same building that houses the courtroom. Rather than crowd the reception area of this floor with clients fresh from the courtroom waiting to make appointments, a detox-acupuncture specialist invites them into a room with fourteen comfortable chairs, where they can "cool

out" and receive acupuncture for stress as well as for detoxification.

Like older drug courts, Midtown Community Court reflects an evolving criminal-justice philosophy which sees
treatment of nonviolent offenders as both cheaper and more
effective than incarceration.

According to Director John Feinblatt, formation of Midtown Community Court was a nearly two-year process, carried out in close consultation with El Río's Ana Oliveira,
who says the court is an aspect of Osborne Treatment Services' La Fuente. Annualized cost of a client going through
any La Fuente program is $750.

15

PRIVATE ACUPUNCTURE TREATMENT FOR ADDICTION

There are about 6,000 licensed professional acupuncturists in the United States, not counting other practitioners who are certified to use acupuncture, such as chiropractors, dentists, medical doctors and osteopaths. It is difficult to determine how many of them treat patients addicted to substances other than tobacco. With the increase in facilities providing NADA-based drug treatment, it is likely that fewer acupuncturists in *solo* private practice treat such clients than did so twenty years ago. However, acupuncture detoxification is a growing presence in private addiction-treatment clinics.

Some people seek private treatment—residential or outpatient—for chemical dependency to protect a job or career. Treatment in private residential settings allows addicted doctors, lawyers, corporate managers and other professionals to keep their problem secret. For those who can afford it, a $12,000, twenty-eight-day rehabilitative program can be camouflaged as a month's vacation in the country.

Others seek private addiction treatment in order to pre-
serve their social comfort. For example, one alcoholic who
had been a varsity athlete at Yale paid to stay at a boxers'
training camp which allowed no liquor, working out with
minor-league fighters for one month a year. His personal
prescription for drying out meshed nicely with denial—he
told friends he just liked to keep fit.

An Ivy League college graduate stopped attending her
AA meeting because, she said later, "My God, I was sitting
next to my butcher!" Recently a similar wealthy suburban
woman with a $2,000 monthly heroin habit said she dropped
out of a municipal hospital outpatient clinic after two weeks
because it was just a block away from where she used to
score before she found a source closer to home. Her other
stated reason was, "I can't relate to street junkies. That was
never my scene."

A look at private clinics indicates that acupuncture has
the same beneficial effects in these settings as in public
clinics. Doug Stellato-Kabat is one of the three directors of
Albany, New York's, Al-Care Outpatient Chemical Dependency Treatment Clinic. His clinic came to use acupuncture
during the course of treating cocaine addicts. At Lowell
Institute (now defunct), which was licensed to do outpatient drug-abuse treatment, he met Ana Oliveira, who lectured there.

Prompted by Oliveira, he looked at the Lincoln program, and proposed acupuncture at Al-Care. A number of
staff members objected to this innovation and quit. But
when the clinic was totally reorganized in 1989, it began to
use the NADA protocol.

Stellato-Kabat prefers working in a private clinic because "you don't have to battle a bureaucracy." While the
chemical dependency treatment field is highly competitive,
he says, few want to treat cocaine users because of the
high relapse rate. Cocaine users are charming, high-energy
people. "The ones I see are also educated and have jobs."

Like other experts, Stellato-Kabat observes that cocaine addiction occurs rapidly, and users tend to seek treatment sooner than do other addicts.

Adolescent addicts of course differ from adults in their social approaches."Teenagers think acupuncture is weird," Kabat says, "and they're highly conservative—have to do what the others do. So one or two being treated by themselves don't do well, but they respond better in a group. Last summer some high-school kids here made it into kind of an in-group."

One licensed acupuncturist serves as a consultant, supervising the work of eleven full-time NADA-trained counselors. The clinic sees 150 clients daily for conventional treatment, and fifteen to twenty for acupuncture. Fifty percent of the clients are self-referred, attracted by other clients' good reports, while others are referred by corporate employee assistance programs, MDs, therapists and lawyers. Ranging in age from fourteen to eighty, 90 percent of the clients are non-Hispanic white, whose socioeconomic status ranges from regular wage-earning through rich and powerful. Forty percent are women. The clinic accepts pregnant women, who are treated for detox with ear-acupuncture.

Al-Care runs a rehabilitative, intensive outpatient program, each day of which includes an hour and a half of therapy and one hour of chemical dependency education, as well as individual and family therapy as needed. At $140 a day, taking into account decreasing frequency of visits following detox, a six-month program costs approximately $6,000, compared to the twelve- to eighteen-thousand dollar, 28-day inpatient program prevailing in 147 drug and alcohol treatment centers surveyed in 1988.✦ Al-Care runs on fees, which are paid by Medicaid, Blue Cross and HMO's.

✦Stan Hart, *Rehab* (New York: HarperCollins, 1988).

Stellato-Kabat stresses the need to fit the program to the client. For example, the clinic has developed separate tracks for gay men and lesbians, among others. A straight woman cocaine user can choose to join either a women's group or a cocaine group.

"Our present cocaine treatment program is working," Stellato-Kabat says. "This NADA protocol is highly effective for cocaine addiction. We're the largest single-site outpatient detox clinic in upstate New York."

Stellato-Kabat, like his counterparts in the public-health sector who use acupuncture for chemical dependency, observes that at first staffers often lack enthusiasm for this treatment. "The field is full of recovering alcoholics who, if they have received only unsophisticated treatment, think AA is revealed truth. I like AA, but there are other ways besides AA. Drug addicts have been through too much to take anything as revelation."

In the course of his work, Stellato-Kabat has observed a cultural change in attitudes toward health care. People recognize that the Western scientific approach is not solving all problems as advertised. A significant clue to this was the establishment in late 1992 of the Office of Alternative Medicine at the National Institutes of Health (NIH). In addition, he finds insurance companies increasingly willing to pay for detox treatment that includes acupuncture, although many still balk at paying for acupuncture itself as a specific billable item. This attitude indicates more progressive thinking than company spokespersons are willing to express on the record: doing so could imply a stated policy of paying for acupuncture across the board. Another reason insurance companies are reticent is that the Food and Drug Administration persists in labeling acupuncture "experimental." A case by case accumulation of documented insurance payments on acupuncture treatment could eventually produce reliable precedents allowing companies to formulate more reasonable policies.

Stellato-Kabat is optimistic about the growth of acupuncture in addiction treatment. There are now three private clinics in the Albany area offering acupuncture detoxification and other acupuncture-based treatment. He points out that "the number of clients here represent a higher percentage of the total population than do those at Lincoln."

Some acupuncturists in private practice treat substance abusers. However, these practitioners tend not to specialize in such clients, and all acupuncturists interviewed on the subject felt that one-on-one treatment might not work so well for chemically dependent people. They also expressed reservations about the single practitioner's ability to serve addicted clients adequately without other supportive therapies in place.

Since the early 1980s, acupuncturists discussing addiction have consistently mentioned Lincoln Detox and NADA. Many practitioners who undertake private treatment of addicts have spent time at Lincoln. Not all, however, have taken the course of training that leads to NADA certification.

One NADA-certified acupuncturist was forced to return to full-time private practice when her rural New England clinic could no longer fund its acupuncture-detox component. Yet she has found that her training and experience continue to serve her well when she treats the occasional chemically-dependent client.

"Detox work is very different from private practice. What goes on in the clinic socially is a major part of how it works. We know how to put needles in—but we learned to focus energy back to the client," she says.

She has taken on one alcoholic—a patient's husband—who said, "If the treatment doesn't work, I'm going out to get drunk." He wanted to be able to blame the acupuncturist if he decided to drink. "But I handed it back to him—told him it sounded pretty boring to spend an evening drunk. What I learned doing NADA work continues to be valuable."

She explains that non-NADA trained acupuncturists often have the impulse to treat general medical problems that present themselves during detox. "Ana [Oliveira] taught us to focus on detox; that must come first," this practitioner says. "It's not as effective if you do general medical during detox. If you start dealing with every little problem, treatment gets diffused."

A midwestern acupuncturist reports that, as in the public programs, very few of his private addiction clients have only one dependency. Cocaine-and-alcohol is a common combination, but there are various others as well. One client was using 92 milligrams of methadone and 60 milligrams of Valium a day as well as heroin, Dilaudid, alcohol, pot, crack and opium when she could get it. It took three months of acupuncture treatment to wean her from this goulash of drugs. Six months later, she was back for more treatment, in the course of which she was functioning adequately and coping with her life while still using "a little" marijuana.

Years ago this acupuncturist served a clinical internship in Hong Kong at Kwong Wah Hospital. He still uses the five-needle method but prefers the earlier system of including some electropotentiation. He also uses symptomatic pulse and tongue diagnosis.

He will treat addicted clients only if they are already seeing a psychotherapist. Experience has shown him that a 12-Step program alone is not enough for his clients. His substance abuse patients are non-Hispanic whites—lawyers, corporate CEO's, etc. Most are men and most have a cocaine habit. Psychiatrists refer their patients to this practitioner and his own clients refer others. Substance abusers are asked to pay in advance for ten sessions, primarily as an incentive to stay in treatment.

People with AIDS/ARC come to this acupuncturist because they've heard of the benefits of acupuncture and Chinese herbal treatment. "I'm very up-front with my clients about the fact that I do treat HIV problems," he explains.

A woman practicing in New York City says that she treats clients for smoking, food problems, alcohol and cocaine abuse with both Chinese herbal medicine and acupuncture.

Chemical dependency treatment, however, does not form a major part of her practice. Her patients' addictions reveal themselves in other ways, some of them psychological: health might be less than optimal, entailing such problems as depression and difficult digestion or interrupted and/or suppressed menstrual periods. This acupuncturist has sometimes found that in treating a condition presented by the patient, she discovers the effects of substance abuse despite the patient's failure to mention it. Her approach is then to ask whether the patient wants to work with her on the addiction problem.

Like her midwestern colleague, she treats some HIV positive people, helping them thrive with herbal medicine. Like other acupuncturists she notes that a sound herbal program benefits the immune system, and treats specific problems within the context of an Oriental medicine view of AIDS. She works with each manifestation as it appears— thrush, diarrhea, etc. She recognizes that many AIDS patients need the strong pharmaceuticals of Western medicine. Treatment is collaborative. She discusses with the patient what improvement or other effects are noted, because some actions of herbal formulations can be incompatible with or counteract some Western drugs.

She has observed HIV-positive people doing well for three or four years without AZT. However, she would never dissuade a person with AIDS from a course of drugs that he or she wishes to continue. Many AIDS patients have a great deal of information about new or promising pharmaceuticals being studied in this country and abroad. "I don't know better than they do," she says.

An East Coast acupuncturist who shares a rural practice with his partner treats people with problems related to tobacco, alcohol and food. He has found that much of what underlies substance abuse also underlies eating disorders.

He concurs with most of the practitioners treating chemical dependency who insist that clients also attend AA meetings. "It is an illusion that you can work it out just by taking treatment from one practitioner."

He mentions people who choose to re-enter the drug culture. The common impression is that relapse into addiction is like having dragged yourself up from quicksand with fingers clutching solid earth, then weakening your grip and sliding back. But this acupuncturist says, "Look at music people in the '60s and '70s, quitting and then doing it again. That, I see as a choice."

Another acupuncturist's experience confirms the evidence that addiction treatment is best done in the context of a program. In a southern capital city, this practitioner treated substance abusers privately in his home-office for several years. He no longer does so. He often found himself working six days a week, and noticed things disappearing from the house.

He tried the prepayment plan, but even addicts who had paid for ten treatments in advance would drop out after a couple of treatments. "Sometimes a person on cocaine would feel better after treatment, then go home and figure, 'I feel pretty good, maybe one snort won't hurt.' " These clients, he says, could be very persuasive people, with the expansive optimism characteristic of a cocaine high.

The physical effects of alcohol abuse appear much later in the patient's history than do those of cocaine. Generally, by the time the alcoholics came to him for treatment, they had such symptoms as DT's, slurred speech and generally visible deterioration.

"What's important about the NADA protocol is that acupuncture shows the addict you can make a difference in how she or he feels."

While maintaining a small private practice, a New York City acupuncturist works part-time at two methadone clinics—one in a municipal hospital, the other freestanding.

Another acupuncturist asked for her help in treating a patient with back pain. The patient was a cocaine user and resisted the idea of being in a group.

When the first acupuncturist treated this coke user she told the second that the client should also go to Cocaine Anonymous (CA) meetings. The client's psychotherapist had been urging the same thing, but the client did not agree to try CA until he heard the advice from all three people involved in his treatment.

"Private treatment is okay," this acupuncturist believes, "if the person has a history, and has gotten clean but sometimes feels cravings." Fundamentally, however, getting clean with other people enables a patient to recognize mutual problems and get support from others, rather than being isolated from them in private treatment.

16

ACUPUNCTURE
AND CIGARETTE SMOKING

The Centers for Disease Control and Prevention's somberly titled *Morbidity and Mortality Weekly Report* of February 1, 1991 reported that 434,175 deaths in 1989 were attributed to smoking. Directly or indirectly this habit causes one of every six deaths. The 1989 Surgeon General's Report identified smoking as a direct cause in 30 percent of cancer deaths—a statistic that includes 87 percent of lung cancer, a major cause of cancer deaths. The report also implicated smoking in 21 percent of coronary heart disease deaths, 18 percent of stroke deaths, and 82 percent of deaths from obstructive pulmonary disease—a category that includes emphysema. Smoking was listed as the *indirect* cause of many other deaths, including those of newborns with low birth weight and other afflictions related to maternal smoking, deaths in cigarette-caused residential fires, and lung cancer deaths of nonsmokers exposed to environmental tobacco smoke.

The Robert Wood Johnson Foundation Report cited in the first chapter of this book, estimates that in 1990, taking into account direct medical expenses, lost work-time due to illness and the value of future lost productivity because of premature death, the total economic cost of smoking in the United States was $72 billion.

Professional acupuncturists in this country provide treatment for smoking control as commonly as they offer general medical treatment for other problems within the scope of practice, e.g., arthritis, asthma, back pain, migraines, weight management and so on. For years acupuncturists have advertised in the Yellow Pages and in newspapers: such ads usually list smoking among the conditions the practitioner treats.

Many people have said that acupuncture was their last resort in trying to quit smoking, and that it worked. Confirmation of this anecdotal evidence has begun to appear, as in a recent Texas report that asserts acupuncture's effectiveness in weaning addicts from cigarettes. Tom Atwood, supervisor of case management, undertook a pilot program for smoking cessation in Waco during 1991 and 1992. Under the auspices of Heart of Texas Region Mental Health and Mental Retardation, sixteen mental patients— each of whom smoked as many as four packs a day and spent 40 to 60 percent of their Public Assistance income on cigarettes—received NADA-based ear acupuncture and supportive counseling. These chronically ill, long-term patients, of whom twelve were schizophrenic, lived in a sixteen-bed group home. They all were actively psychotic, and a step away from psychiatric-hospital admission.

After a year of acupuncture and supportive counseling, four of the patients had quit smoking, two smoked on and off, eight had decreased their smoking by 40 percent and two still smoked as much as ever. Group members spent a total of $6,000 less on cigarettes than they had the previous year. As of January 1994, smoking-cessation statistics for this group remained the same.

An unforeseen by-product of the Waco study was that group members were admitted to psychiatric hospitals much less often than before—pre-acupuncture admissions averaged one every forty-six days. Post-acupuncture, this rate dropped to one every 604 days. The acupuncture treatment thus was doubly cost effective, reducing the money spent on cigarettes, and reducing hospital admissions.

Public-sector acupuncture-based substance abuse programs developed for illegal drug and alcohol users who come under control of public agencies and institutions—or are at risk of being under such control—also reveal acupuncture's value in treating tobacco addiction. Clients in such programs often report a decline in cigarette smoking, a beneficial side effect of treatment for the *primary* drug of abuse.

"Who, me? An addict? I don't even drink. Just because I smoke a pack a day . . . I know I should quit, but *addiction*—that's something else!" Not true: cigarette smoking exhibits the primary criteria of drug addiction as listed in the 1988 Surgeon General's Report:

"Highly controlled or compulsive pattern of drug use. Pyschoactive or mood-altering effects involved in pattern of drug taking. Drug functioning as reinforcer to strengthen behavior and lead to further drug ingestion."

At a time when few deny that heroin, cocaine and alcohol are addictive, a profound cultural bias still makes it hard for smokers to admit that their habit is on a par with addiction to these other drugs.

"Be nonchalant, light a Murad", said a 1920s advertising slogan. In mid-century, "I'd walk a mile for a Camel" was a huckster's fantasy based on reality: many a heavy smoker has slogged twenty blocks through a storm at midnight to buy a pack of cigarettes. For decades cigarette smoking was not only acceptable to mainstream society, but also a rite of passage for teenagers who emulated adult sophistication as portrayed by movie heroines and heroes, whose every important screen moment was punctuated by lighting or sharing a cigarette. As advertising became more complex, cigarettes were even sold as the key to sexual identity, with the Marlboro Man riding tall in the saddle while the Virginia Slims ads shouted "You've come a long way baby" to the liberated modern woman.

The fifty years in which cigarette smoking became thoroughly intertwined with our social fabric afforded smokers no preparation for the 1964 Surgeon General's Report on Smoking and Health. The Report, prepared by an advisory committee for Surgeon General Luther L. Terry, was released at a Saturday morning press conference. Journalists were sequestered, given an hour and a half to read the report, and allowed no access to telephones until after the question-and-answer session. Knowing the tobacco industry's extensive involvement in American business, planners chose a Saturday in order to avoid a drastic stockmarket upset in the wake of what they suspected would become one of the year's top news stories.

The 1964 report described cigarette smoking as "habituating." Fifteen years later, the 1979 report called smoking "the prototypical substance abuse dependency." The 1988 report focused entirely on tobacco use as addiction, declaring:

"1. Cigarettes and other forms of tobacco are addicting.

"2. Nicotine is the drug in tobacco that causes addiction.

"3. The pharmacological and behavioral processes that determine tobacco addiction are similar to those that determine addiction to drugs such as heroin or cocaine."

At the consumer level, it is noteworthy that clinical information packaged with Nicoderm,✦ a nicotine patch sold by prescription only, includes this passage: "Withdrawal from nicotine by addicted individuals is characterized by craving, nervousness, restlessness, irritability, mood lability, anxiety, drowsiness, sleep disturbances, impaired concentration, increased appetite, minor somatic complaints (headache, myalgia, constipation, fatigue), and weight gain."

✦1992, Marion Merrell Dow, Inc.

It may be almost impossible for those who never smoked to understand the cigarette habit's death-grip on dedicated users. The following anecdotes show the difficulty of freeing oneself from a compulsive activity that touches all aspects of daily life.

A fifty-one-year-old California journalist discussed his habit. "In college and the army, we'd eat something, drink something, and smoke. You'd smoke enough to keep the fix going. After that, it depends. I went from one pack a day to two. I got a craving even at the movies; that's only two hours. If they'd had the no-smoking rule on transcontinental flights, I don't know what I would have done. You see smokers now lighting up in the jetway when they come off the plane."

At forty, he tried to quit cold turkey. During the first week he fished butts from his fireplace and from ashtrays. Then he really quit. For a year he felt symptoms—headaches, insomnia and irritability—and craving. Most of that time he was reporting on trials. "It was okay in the courtroom; you never smoked there anyway. But when court recessed, all the reporters rushed out to the hall to light up. I chewed my fingernails nearly to the elbow. Even now, eleven years later, about once a week I feel a psychological craving; I really want a cigarette. It's not physiological. But if I lit one, I'd be right back doing two packs a day."

A year after he quit, the journalist had a massive heart attack. Doctors told him the year of not smoking was crucial to his survival.

[P]rolonged ingestion of nicotine leads to tolerance, a tendency to consume increasing amounts of a drug, presumably to achieve a desired euphoric or other effect. Prolonged use also leads to physical dependence, as indexed by various psychological and physical withdrawal symptoms following cessation of smoking, (1989 Surgeon General's Report).

A forty-year-old Montana businesswoman, racecar driver and 25-year smoker has tried several times to break her pack-a-day habit. She says she doesn't want her young children to be exposed to so much smoke, and she wants to be alive and vigorous when they grow up.

Heavy smoking is normal in her small town. Her husband smokes two packs a day. She tried using a mail order motivational tape, packaged with "some kind of pills," she says, but that technique was not helpful. A dreadfully bitter prescription chewing gum was helpful, but not effective enough to counter her response to being with heavy smokers. Recently she quit cold turkey and began a daily aerobics class. After six weeks she resumed smoking. Summarizing her limited success she says, "You're going along fine, and then there's a pebble in the road. You stumble and find yourself back where you started."

[T]he basis for nicotine addiction rests on the interaction of conditioning processes and nicotine action in the brain, (1989 Surgeon General's Report).

A seventy-year-old New York theater director insists it was not the nicotine but the ritual that kept him smoking more than two packs a day without ever really enjoying cigarettes. "I hated smoking. It was a nuisance never going anywhere without first checking to see that I had cigarettes. It was a burden. I'd light one while waiting for rehearsals to start, when talking to the actors, when rehearsal broke, waiting for an elevator, when I got out of the elevator, waiting for the red light to change crossing the street, when I made a phone call or answered the phone—you name it."

This man was forced to quit. "I remember lighting a cigarette and feeling sick in a strange way. I put the cigarette out, called my doctor, and he met me in the emergency room. I was in the ICU for 24 hours. I still remember the fear. I've never even thought of smoking in the twelve years since my heart attack."

Smoking is continued despite a desire to quit, (1989 Surgeon General's Report).

A chain-smoking retired professional dancer now in her mid-sixties saw her mother die of cigarette-induced emphysema some twenty years ago. Ten years after her mother's death the retired dancer had a cancerous part of one lung removed. After six weeks she began to smoke again. Recently, for a complex assortment of health problems, she spent time in an iron lung, and remarked to her (non-smoking) daughters, "See what it took to make me quit?"

Smoking is continued . . . in many cases, despite clear harm to the individual, (1989 Surgeon General's Report).

A former Lincoln Detox patient and longtime Lincoln Acupuncture Clinic staff member tells how she successfully quit smoking. "Since I was seventeen, I smoked three packs a day. I'd be treating people and running out to grab a smoke." She had one treatment—press needles left overnight in the ears at Lung point. Since then she has had about five treatments at varying intervals. Each treatment entailed wearing press needles for a day at a time. She has been a nonsmoker for eleven years.

The Lincoln staffer and the California journalist made intellectual decisions. She found it absurd to be treating addicts while gripped by her own need for tobacco. He had a family history of heart attacks and also responded to the prevailing awareness that smoking is unhealthy. Like most who eventually succeed in becoming nonsmokers, the Montana racer oscillates between quitting and relapsing. The New York director remains happy that he was eventually jolted out of his smoking habit. The former dancer denied the danger she courted. People with less dramatic health conditions than hers tolerate worsening asthma, chronic bronchitis, cardiac difficulties or migraines rather than give up cigarettes.

Studies indicating a correlation between higher education levels and quitting suggest that the cigarette smoker's image has come a long way—from debonair to downscale.

Although breaking the cigarette habit shares characteristics with struggles to give up alcohol or illegal drugs, no agency can order smokers to seek treatment. The desperate would-be nonsmoker is unlikely to enroll in a public-health, acupuncture-based substance abuse program. Consequently most acupuncture treatments for nicotine dependence are given in private practice.

Smokers' patterns—cues for lighting up—and rationales for smoking vary tremendously, as do the aftereffects of quitting. One patient who had previously smoked three packs a day told an acupuncturist, "In the waiting room was the first time I've spent a waking hour without lighting one cigarette from another." One person gains weight after giving up cigarettes, while another loses weight because she no longer snacks to remove the bad taste of tobacco from her mouth. One person quits, and a year later smokes a cigarette but feels no urge to have another. Someone else quits. Three years later, under stress, he resumes smoking, and within days is back to his previous multi-pack level.

There is no single standard acupuncture formula for nicotine addiction. Treatment varies according to the practitioner's style, training, and diagnosis of the individual patient. In an article titled "The Treatment of Smoking and Nicotine Addiction with Acupuncture," senior acupuncturist Stuart Kutchins emphasizes the importance of enlisting the patient's active cooperation in setting up a program to support the difficult task of quitting.*

---

*The Clinical Management of Nicotine Dependence, edited by James A. Cocores, MD (New York: Springer Verlag, 1991).

Acupuncture alone cannot do the job. The smoker must engage will power in the effort, and the most effective treatment involves an alliance between the acupuncturist and the client. A reasonable respect for the client accepts a smoker's view that there are some positive aspects to the use of cigarettes. As noted in the 1989 Surgeon General's Report, "Nicotine . . . can serve to reduce anxiety or produce euphoria and enhance vigilance for certain cognitive tasks." Acupuncture, too, reduces anxiety and induces a sense of well-being and clearmindedness—but only experience proves this to the would-be nonsmoker.

Some acupuncturists begin with needling at earpoints, selecting from combinations of Shen Men, Sympathetic, Kidney and Liver according to the Lincoln/NADA detox formula. Usually a week or two after detox, they initiate treatment at body points appropriate to the individual client's physiological and behavioral responses. According to one acupuncturist, "The ear is where you deal with the drug. You treat the person by using body points."

Others use ear points and traditional body points concurrently. An acupuncturist with many years in urban practice sees about twelve patients every week who wish to rid themselves of cigarette habits ranging from half a pack to three packs per day. He treats the client twice a week for two to three weeks, selecting ear points from Stomach, Lung, Heart, Liver, Kidney, and Shen Men and body points when appropriate. His observation is that nobody ever quits permanently after one visit, and he feels that advertisements suggesting a quick fix do a disservice to the acupuncture profession. He has seen clients do well with one course of treatment, but more often, after months or years, the urge may reappear. A client who takes a second course of treatment is usually successful in remaining a nonsmoker. This practitioner's observation confirms many of his colleagues': acupuncture paves the way to becoming a nonsmoker in the critical withdrawal phase, but motivation is important and the client must be prepared to return for an additional course of treatment if cravings return.

Combining Eastern and Western medicine, another practitioner recommends supplemental Chinese medicine–based herbal formulas to support lung energy as well as vitamin supplements. He advises avoiding tea, coffee, alcohol and excessive sweet foods. He warns that spicy and fatty foods tend to excite craving. At half his usual fee he gives a smoke-ending program every fall in conjunction with a local anti-smoking campaign in Colorado. The program includes four treatments the first week, a week without treatment, then one more treatment—two if needed. Patients may also use a Chinese herbal drink called West Lake Stop Smoking Tea, taking two to three cups a day and another cup when there is an overwhelming urge to smoke. The tea contains lotus seed, ginseng leaf, lucid [shiny] asparagus, betel nut and licorice root.

The alliance between practitioner and client may be quite simple in practice. For instance, one acupuncturist requires patients to toss their cigarettes into the office wastebasket before he inserts needles. He gives a five-treatment course in which two press-needles are inserted alongside the tragus of one ear the first week, and of the other ear the next. The patient is instructed to rub the tape-covered needles if craving occurs.

Asking his patients for still more effort and preparation, another acupuncturist uses a form of gradual withdrawal, telling the two-pack-a-day smoker, "You'll do better if you're down to a pack a day before we start treatment. The way to do that is to remove one cigarette from the pack and throw it away. The next day, you remove two, and so forth." Patients, he says, learn to stretch out the time between cigarettes. By the time they begin treatment, they not only know they are able to reduce nicotine intake; but they have experienced enough nicotine deprivation that the first acupuncture session gives strong relief from craving. This initial relief is a great inducement to complete the course of treatment.

Some acupuncturists ask patients to analyze the cues that induce them to smoke in the course of a typical day. These cues include emotional, environmental and other triggers. This approach is akin to that of diet programs which make participants list everything they eat for a week before beginning the regimen.

Still another acupuncturist with a high success rate is selective about the clients he takes. Those he accepts after an initial consultation including a detailed psychosocial questionnaire—for which a fee is charged—must feel as if they've made the "varsity cut." It is an encouraging incentive to begin the difficult work of quitting.

Stuart Kutchins writes, "While long-range outcomes may reflect more on the characteristics of the client and the whole treatment program, middle-range (second stage) outcomes are important to consider, as many apparent successes recidivate in the transition from withdrawing to stably recovered if there is inadequate follow-through. This second stage may be considered to begin at the close of withdrawal, in one to two weeks after the last cigarette was smoked, and to end at the time when the client no longer feels that she or he confronts nonsmoking as a difficult or unresolved issue."

Many acupuncturists receive referrals of doctors' patients who fail to comply with the prescription to stop smoking. As has been shown, acupuncture's effectiveness in weaning people from cigarettes is well accepted. But success rates only improve to the degree that acupuncture is part of an entire holistic treatment package tailored to the client's smoking profile.

17

THE DURABLE ESTABLISHMENT

New York City Health and Hospitals Corporation
Lincoln Medical & Mental Health Center
Department of Psychiatry
Substance Abuse Division

With its plain blue and red letters on a white background, the new sign over the doorway to the gray brick building is more formal than the old blue and orange one. A guard is still at the desk as visitors enter and explain their business before proceeding through the terrazzo-floored lobby to the acupuncture room. Two computer monitors now stand prominently on the desk at the entrance to the treatment room. The same green chairs are there and the place seems unchanged except by time, which has brought new faces. The work-style persists, friendly, low-key, calm, unhurried. Most of the chairs are occupied by men and women with needles protruding from their ears. As always, it is an extraordinarily tranquil scene.

But for all its tranquility, this room has for twenty years been the source of transformational energy that has spread to other places. From its difficult birth as Lincoln Detox, this clinic has grown into the recognized center of acupuncture-based addiction treatment on an outpatient basis. Lincoln Acupuncture Clinic continues its daily work of treating, teaching and advocating, while the treatment model initiated here in the South Bronx is disseminated nationally and internationally.

Having passed through the pioneer stage, acupuncture-based programs now proliferate, forming a second wave. The National Acupuncture Detoxification Association's methods maintain a valid life of their own even after the departure of those who originally introduced these methods to any one region.

Texas, for example, lost three prominent NADA workers, yet programs expand and their numbers continue to increase. With state funding, a Houston hospital undertook a study comparing acupuncture with medication in treating substance abuse. The program's original acupuncturist was Father Mark Pemberton, whose meticulous arrangements allowed the program to continue seamlessly after his death in the summer of 1992. As mentioned earlier, in Waco, the county mental health system used NADA methods in a pilot program which successfully reduced rehospitalization in a group of chronic mental patients.

NADA, the outgrowth of Lincoln Acupuncture Clinic, is not monolithic. Different regional circumstances make local entities a logical development. State NADAs have been formed in California, Connecticut and Texas. Quality control is maintained by a collective agreement that training for potential practitioners requires seventy hours: twenty-four hours of didactic instruction, six hours of exposure to 12-Step programs and forty hours of supervised apprenticeship. NADA certification requires that candidates be recommended for training, and results be approved by trainers and by a regional or national board member. Geography and environment affect the design of training sessions. New York State law exempts from normal licensing acupuncture conducted in a state-approved drug or alcohol treatment program, provided that clinicians receive proper training and supervision. With senior staff member Carlos Alvarez as primary instructor, Lincoln's Acupuncture Training Institute trained 2,000 clinicians from 1991–1995. The institute's waiting list is three months long. Its urban location and large clinic size make it possible to combine instruction and apprenticeship in one location. In some regions it is more convenient to arrange weekend training sessions with apprenticeship at a local clinic under supervision of a NADA-trained, licensed acupuncturist.

Quality control with flexibility allows NADA programs to function well in England, France, Germany, Hungary, Nepal, Saudi Arabia, Spain, Sweden and Trinidad.

NADA groups have been formed in Germany, Great Britain, Hungary and Sweden. (They all use NADA in their identifying names, even though the word originally applied to the U.S. national organization.)

John Tindall conducts a weekly Chinese medicine group at Phoenix House London. This may have repercussions in the United States, where the original United States Phoenix House organization does not sanction the use of detox acupuncture.

In Hungary, 25 percent of the adult population is alcoholic. Hungarian NADA, coordinated by acupuncturist Paul Zmiewski, who moved to Budapest in the winter of 1991/ 1992, developed rapidly. Fifteen treatment programs were established in the first year. Zmiewski had begun a similar process of providing NADA training sessions in Poland, Romania and Russia before he died in September 1993. The following year Brian McKenna moved to Budapest to carry on the NADA work. During his first year McKenna trained 283 individuals in the NADA protocol.

In the summer of 1995, the Soros Foundation—already a major contributor to NADA/Hungary—announced ongoing funding which fully supports this acupuncture work, including acupuncture-detox training for Eastern Europe as well as Hungary. By January 1996, McKenna will have trained 10 NADA *trainers,* each based in his or her own clinic: 6 in Hungary, 2 in Romania, and 2 in Slovakia.

The NADA protocol is being used in methadone maintenance programs. While this contemporary application of acupuncture to methadone users harks back to the origins of Lincoln Detox, the clients have different habits. The population of old-fashioned heroin-only addicts, for whom methadone was originally designed, is in decline. They are aging out of society, and some are in nursing homes which arrange their outpatient treatment at various facilities. Nowadays many methadone patients also use cocaine and alcohol, among other auxiliary substances. As one client says, "If you're on the methadone program you don't get much from the dope [heroin], so you add a little coke, to give it something."

Clinically, acupuncture has proven effective in reducing these methadone users' secondary addictions. On the research front, Yale University's successful pilot program using acupuncture to reduce methadone clients' secondary cocaine addiction confirms clinical experience. Acupuncture reduces cravings for cocaine, alcohol and other substances. It alleviates the anxiety and aggressive behavior often seen in methadone clients. This is a boon to clinics, freestanding or hospital-based, as it cuts down disruptive behavior and thus helps make the clinic run more smoothly. Also, with time, acupuncture allows reduction of dosage. This last effect is obviously not the primary goal for methadone clinics public or private, as a clinic needs a full supply of clients in order to continue its existence. However, clinics using a variety of therapies to treat chemical dependency are apt to welcome acupuncture-induced dosage reduction. In mid-1995, as an outgrowth of the Yale acupuncture-methadone studies, the Center on Addiction and

Substance Abuse (CASA) received a $3.5 million research grant, half from the Conrad Hilton Foundation, the balance from several federal government agencies. The money will support acupuncture research conducted by Herb Cleaver who for 25 years was professor of Psychiatry at Yale; and during whose tenure Yale carried out research on heroin, cocaine and alcohol addiction.

Since the mid-1960s changing times have compelled law enforcement agencies to begin sharing control over drug addiction solutions. Increasingly chemical dependency has also become the domain of public-health medicine and of social-welfare agencies. These three powerful, turf-concious entities are not born allies, but today many authorities in the three fields agree enthusiastically on the effectiveness of acupuncture-based treatment. Now pilot programs based on the Lincoln model show the way to saving billions of public-health, criminal justice and social welfare dollars.

The acupuncture needle—small and cheap—is proving the most powerful weapon in the real war on drugs—the fight to curb addiction by transforming lives.

BIBLIOGRAPHY

Ackerman, Ruth. *Acupuncture Treatment of Chemical Dependency: A Review of the Literature.* Vancouver, Wash.: NADA Literature Clearinghouse, 1995.

Blum, Robert W., MD, Brian Harmon, Linda Harris, Lois Bergeisen and Michael Resnick. "Native American Indian–Alaska Youth Health," *Journal of the American Medical Association* 267, no. 12 (March 25, 1992).

Brewington, V., M. Smith, and D. Lipton. "Acupuncture as a Detoxification Treatment: An Analysis of Controlled Research," *Journal of Substance Abuse Treatment, 11, no. 4, pages 289-307, 1994.*

Brumbaugh, Alex G. *Transformation & Recovery: A Guide for the Design & Development of Acupuncture-Based Chemical Dependency Treatment Programs.* Santa Barbara, Calif.: Stillpoint Press, 1994.

Bullock, Milton L., Andrew J. Umen, Patricia D. Culliton and Robert T. Olander. "Acupuncture Treatment of Alcoholic Recidivism: A Pilot Study," *Alcoholism: Clinical & Experimental Research* 11, no. 3 (May–June 1987).

Falco, Mathea. *The Making of a Drug-Free America: Programs That Work.* New York: Times Books, 1992.

Fogelman, Betsy, ed. *The Oriental Medicine Resource Guide: An Informal Sourcebook.* InWord Press, 1993. (Includes list of twenty-seven NADA-based programs in eight states.)

Goh, Magnolia, and Zhaoling Tang. *Alternative Treatments for HIV Infection.* New York: Science Press, 1995.

Hart, Stan. *Rehab.* New York: HarperCollins, 1988.

Horgan, Constance, et al. *Substance Abuse: The Nation's Number One Health Problem.* Princeton, New Jersey: Robert Wood Johnson Foundation, 1993.

Kutchins, Stuart. "The Treatment of Smoking and Nicotine Addiction with Acupuncture." In *The Clinical Management of Nicotine Dependence* edited by James A. Cocores. New York: Springer Verlag, 1991.

McWilliams, John C. *The Protectors: Harry J. Anslinger and the Federal Bureau of Narcotics, 1930–1962.* Carlbury, New Jersey: Associated University Presses, 1990.

NADA (National Acupuncture Detoxification Association) Literature Clearinghouse. Anecdotal reports from practicing clinicians; reprints of scientific papers from journals; audiotapes and videotapes on clinical practice. This material is the officially accepted body of knowledge from the NADA board. To receive list of titles send a self-addressed, stamped envelope to: NADA Literature Clearinghouse, P.O. Box 1927, Vancouver, WA 98668.

Needham, Joseph, and Gwei-Dje Lu. *Celestial Lancets: A History and Rationale of Acupuncture and Moxibustion.* Cambridge: Cambridge University Press, 1980.

Nordenström, Bjorn. *Biologically Closed Electric Circuits: Clinical and Theoretical Evidence for an Additional Circulatory System.* Stockholm: Nordic Medical Publications, 1983.

Olsen, Terry. *International Handbook of Ear Reflex Points.* Los Angeles: Health Care Alternatives, 1995.

Omura, Yoshiaki. *Acupuncture Medicine.* Tokyo: Japan Publications, 1980.

Parson, Ann. "Getting the Point," *Harvard Health Letter* 18, no. 10 (August 1993).

Pomerantz, Bruce, MD. *FDA testimony, transcript,* 1991. Available from American Association of Acupuncture and Oriental Medicine, 433 Front Street, Carasauqua, PA 18032.

Renaud, Jay, ed. *Guidepoints: Acupuncture in Recovery.* Independent monthly newsletter for professionals "concerned with innovative treatment of addictive and mental disorders." (Emphasizes funding, public policy, science and clinical practice.) Subscription: $180 per year. Order from: J & M Reports, 7402 NE 58th Street, Vancouver, WA 98662.

Ryan, Mary Kay and Arthur D. Shattuck. *Treating AIDS With Chinese Medicine.* Berkeley, Calif.: Pacific View Press, 1994.

Simmons, Boyd. "Alcohol, The Legal Drug," *National Geographic* (February 1992). (Includes sidebar on "Fetal Alcohol Syndrome" by George Steinmetz.)

Smith, Michael O., MD, D.Ac., Khunat Ra and Ana Oliviera. *Acupuncture Treatment for Alcoholism.* New York: Lincoln Hospital Substance Abuse Division, 1986.

De Vernejoul, Pierre, Pierre Albarede and Jean Claude Darras. "Investigation of Acupuncture Meridians by Radioactive Tracers." *Bulletin of the National Academy of Medicine* (Paris) 169, no. 7 (1985).

Also available from Pacific View Press

TREATING AIDS WITH CHINESE MEDICINE
by Mary Kay Ryan and Arthur D. Shattuck

This comprehensive handbook is the first to systematically present an overall framework for understanding and treating HIV disease from the perspective of traditional Chinese medicine. Based on the authors' extensive clinical experience, it provides effective herbal and acupuncture strategies for addressing the AIDS milieu of illness, infection, and drug side effects.

Paper, $29.95, ISBN 1-881896-07-2

CHINESE BODYWORK
A COMPLETE HANDBOOK OF
CHINESE THERAPEUTIC MASSAGE
Edited by Sun Chengnan

Massage is an integral part of traditional Chinese healing arts. Based in meridian theory, it promotes the circulation of vital energy and blood, regulating the function of the meridians, and internal organs to improve vitality and restore health. *Chinese Bodywork,* incorporating the experience of over a dozen of China's leading practitioners, is sure to become the standard for students of traditional Chinese medicine.

Cloth, $50.00, ISBN 1-881896-06-4

ACUPUNCTURE, MERIDIAN THEORY, AND ACUPUNCTURE POINTS
by Li Ding

Professor Li Ding presents a lucid, organized approach to the fundamental concepts that practitioners of traditional Chinese medicine must master.

Cloth, $60.00, 0-8351-2143-7

CHINA
BUSINESS STRATEGIES FOR THE '90S
by Arne J. de Keijzer

This excellent resource draws on the experiences of companies over the past 15 years to carefully identify the lessons learned and the implications for anyone contemplating business with China. Also ideal for courses on international law and business, and for anyone looking at China's economy, international relations, or development strategy.

Paper, $24.95, 1-881896-00-5

VIETNAM
BUSINESS OPPORTUNITIES AND RISKS
by Joseph P. Quinlan

A concise guide to one of the world's hottest new markets, offering a quick, comprehensive snapshot of the country. It identifies the key variables that must be considered by anyone doing business. The author provides analysis as well as practical information on laws, forms of foreign investment, taxes, and investment regulations.

Paper, $19.95, 1-881896-10-2

CHINA ON THE EDGE
CRISIS OF ECOLOGY AND DEVELOPMENT
by He Bochuan

One of China's leading futurists paints a disturbing picture of the environmental situation and the problems of development in his country. His thesis is that overpopulation and the demands of a growing economy are placing China on the brink of an environmental disaster. This highly detailed account of the challenges facing China is required reading for the economic and political decision makers of the West.

Paper, $16.95, 0-8351-2448-7

TEACHING ENGLISH IN ASIA
FINDING A JOB AND DOING IT WELL
by Galen Harris Valle

This book aims to provide the information needed to work as a teacher in China, Japan, Indonesia, Thailand, Korea, and other Asian countries. It is addressed to travelers—those who seek to combine their interest in Asia with the skills necessary to live and work there, and to teachers—those with previous training or experience who want to learn how to best use these skills with Asian students.

Paper, $19.95, 1-881896-11-0

RED EGGS AND DRAGON BOATS
CELEBRATING CHINESE FESTIVALS
by Carol Stepanchuk

This beautiful book shares the experience of four of China's major festivals, celebrated by Chinese people throughout the world, plus a traditional welcoming party for a new baby with readers from 8 to 12. Stories, folklore, customs, and recipes for holiday treats are accompanied by wonderful illustrations of festival activities, painted by some of China's best folk artists.

Cloth, $16.95, 1-881896-08-0

LONG IS A DRAGON
CHINESE WRITING FOR CHILDREN
by Peggy Goldstein

A Parents' Choice Award-winning introduction to the Chinese writing system, which takes the reader stroke by stroke from the pictographs of ancient times to the characters of today. Written for children ages 8 to 12, this book includes over 75 characters, including the number system.

Cloth, $15.95, 1-881896-01-3

For a complete catalog, write:
Pacific View Press
P. O. Box 2657
Berkeley, CA 94702